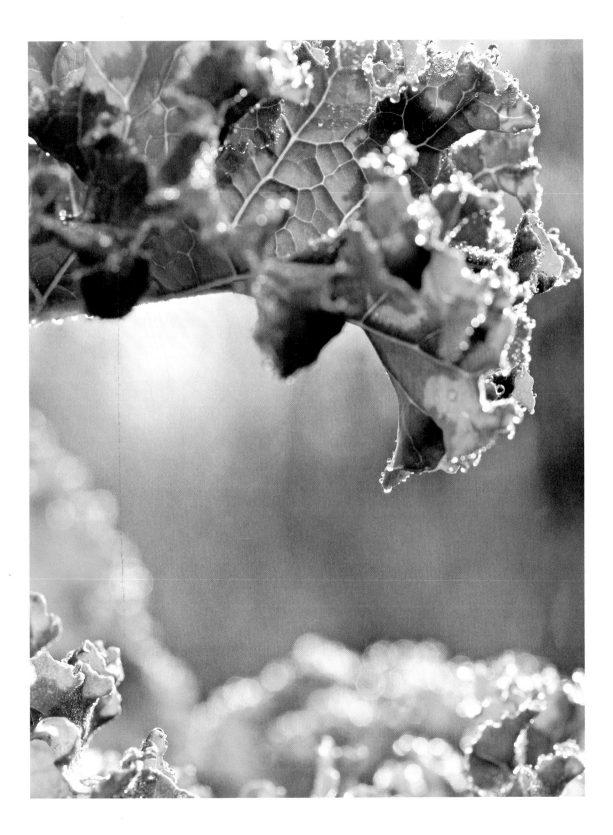

FIFTY SHADES OF *Kale*

FIFTY SHADES OF *Kale*

50 FRESH AND SATISFYING RECIPES THAT ARE BOUND TO PLEASE

Drew Ramsey, M.D., & Jennifer Iserloh

With photographs by Ian McSpadden

HARPER WAVE

An Imprint of HarperCollins*Publishers*

www.harpercollins.com

HarperCollins books may be purchased for educational, business, or sales promotional use. For information, please write: Special Markets Department, HarperCollins Publishers, 10 East 53rd Street, New York, NY 10022.

Photographs © Ian McSpadden

FIRST EDITION

Book Design by Leah Carlson-Stanisic

Library of Congress Cataloging-in-Publication Data is available upon request.

ISBN: 978-0-06-227288-1

13 14 15 16 17 OV/RRD 10 9 8 7 6 5 4 3 2 1

To our muse and mistress, Kale.

May she seduce and satisfy you.

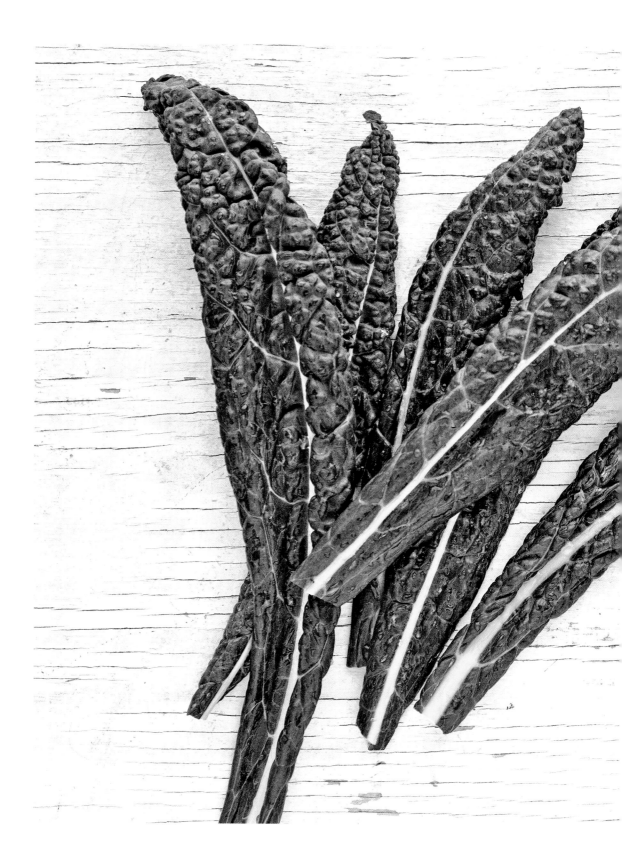

Contents

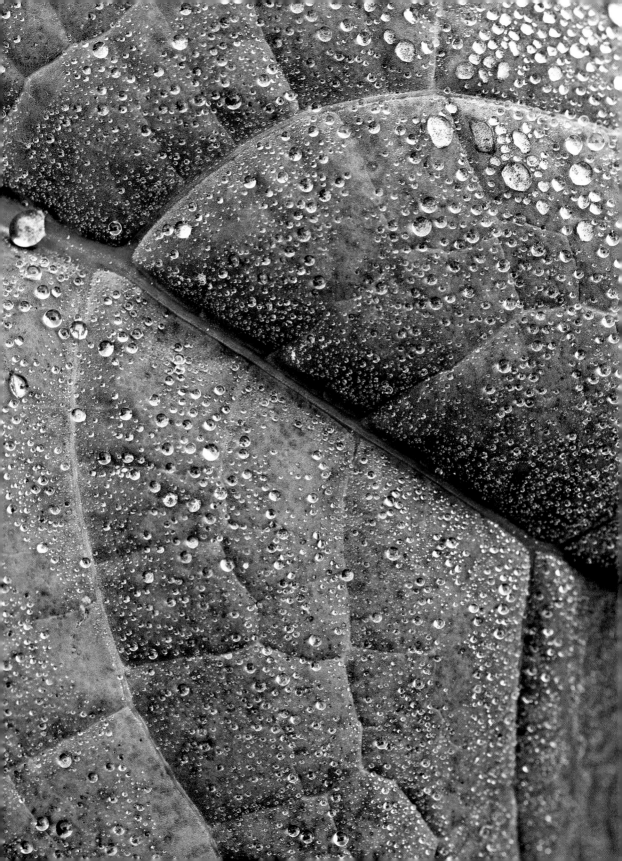

Introduction

*N*othing is sexier than a sharp, happy mind atop a lean, healthy body. Few foods are able to deliver this promise like kale. She is the ideal plant in many ways: hardy and easy to grow, nutrient dense, and delicious.

Kale is the queen of the cruciferous vegetables, a family of superfoods packed with nutritional benefits. She delivers a huge dose of vitamin K* (with more than 600 percent of your daily allowance per serving), and plays a starring role in supporting brain and bone health.

She offers more vitamin C than an orange, more pro-vitamin A than any other leafy green, and a tiny one-cup serving has close to three times as much calcium as a school lunch–size carton of milk. The fats are in perfect ratio— in fact the main source of fat in kale is omega-3 fat, which is essential for optimum health. With just one cup, kale brings a whopping 121 mg of the core omega-3, alpha-linoleic acid (ALA), to the table.

But it is her lesser-known qualities that enchant and hold us prisoner. In addition to offering a bounty of vitamins and minerals, kale possesses a veritable medicine chest of healthy molecules known as phytonutrients. These plant-based molecules travel from the end of your fork to the very center of your cells, where they turn on genes that boost your body's natural ability to

---

* If you take blood thinners like warfarin, or have a blood clotting disorder, speak with your doctor before you begin to eat kale regularly. Vitamin K can interfere with some anticlotting medications. Also, some people with thyroid sensitivity may react to molecules called goitrogens that are found in kale, though these molecules do break down when kale is cooked.

detox. The sulforaphane in kale helps to protect against diseases like cancer and diabetes. Her flavonoids—responsible for her many deep colors—offer a boost to cardiac health and your immune system.

Ultimately, this book aims to release you from the bondage of guilt—to encourage you to prepare and eat decadent-tasting foods that are also good for you. Kale not only offers a wide array of health benefits, it also helps you to stay lean. At only 33 calories per cup, kale offers a lot of nutrient value for very few calories. And because the nutrients in kale become more bioavailable (able to be absorbed and utilized by your body) when paired with other specific nutrients, you'll find that you can indulge in foods you might typically consider sinful. The recipes in this book will show you how to cook with ingredients like butter, eggs, red meat, and pasta in a healthy manner. So whether you're a cooking novice and want to start with a one-day love affair or a real kale submissive, you will undoubtedly succumb to her charms. And with fifty kale-centric recipes, like Hot Bacon Kale, Spicy Mussels with Kale, and Kale and Black Cherry Sorbet . . . resistance is futile.

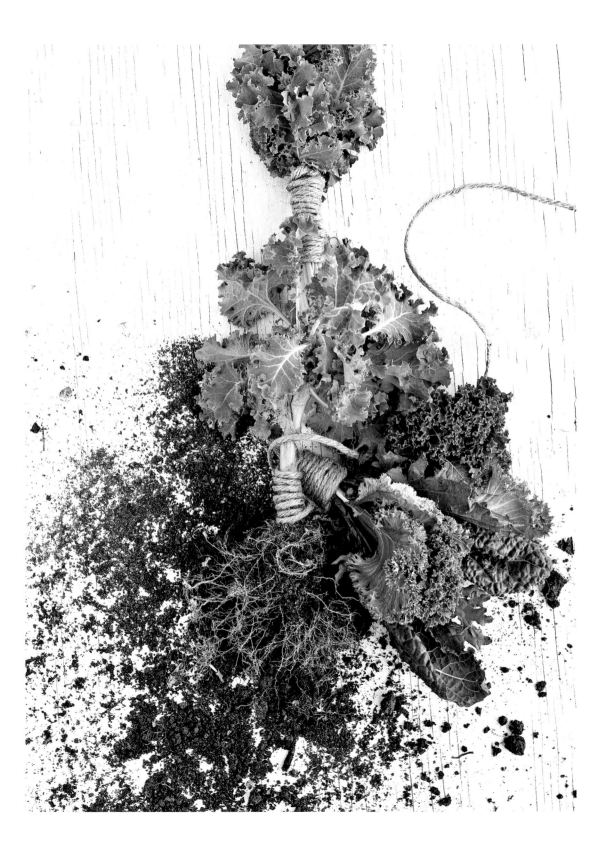

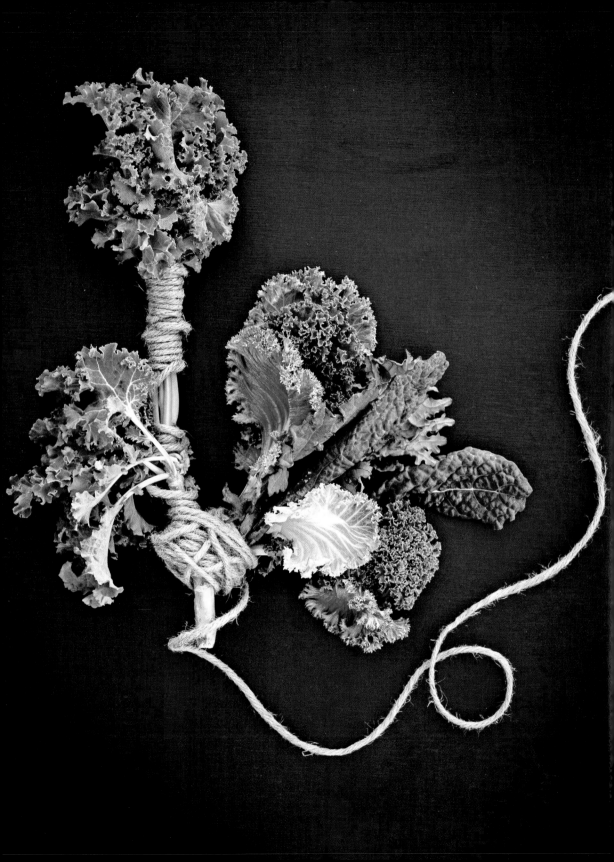

1.

Submit to Her

Charms

*T*he best sensual relationships require discipline to thrive. When it comes to cooking with kale, it's important to treat her with respect, and to pair her with the best-quality ingredients you are able to find, such as grass-fed beef and eggs from pasture-raised hens. Just like anything truly sexy, these fifty recipes are both exciting and tasteful. If you are ready to be turned on to the healthier, sexier you, here are a few guidelines to help you maximize the benefits (and flavor) of kale.

➤ Try to use *organic* kale whenever possible. Kale was recently added to the Environmental Working Group's "Dirty Dozen" list of vegetables most likely to contain

pesticides (see page 11), so it's worth the extra expense to buy organic.

➤ Treat your kale with care. Despite her hearty exterior, kale is tender and fragile. Don't leave her out on

- the countertop or prewash her too far in advance—nobody likes a limp vegetable.
- Store your kale in the crisper, loosely gathered in a plastic bag. Add a paper towel or wrap her in a dry paper towel to trap excess moisture and keep her fresher and fuller longer.
- Don't overcook your kale. Not only will the taste and texture suffer from overexposure to heat, but she will lose some of her nutrient value if cooked for too long. As a rule of thumb, ten minutes is the maximum amount of time you want to expose kale to direct heat. For pan cooking, use a small metal lid to gently press down the kale as you turn it.

Fifty Shades of Kale

*O*K, so it's not quite *fifty* . . . but kale does come close to offering fifty shades of variety. Cornell University lists forty-eight known kale varietals providing you with a vast world of kale to explore. From deep purples and vibrant greens to translucent whites and radiant pinks, all are members of the cruciferous vegetable family, which includes other so-called superfoods like broccoli, bok choy, and Brussels sprouts.

All crucifers evolved from cabbage and thus all bear the same scientific name, *Brassica oleracea*. Kale belongs to the Acephala group of crucifers, literally meaning "no head," as, unlike cabbage and broccoli, kale leaves aren't formed around a central head.

Each variety of kale offers unique flavor notes, color, and texture. Here is a brief overview of the varieties that are used in the recipes in this book. These are some of the most common varietals and should be easy to find at the grocery store or at your local farmers' markets.

Curly Green

This is the classic varietal that most people think of when they hear the word *kale*. It's also probably the most common one found in your grocery store. With curly leaves and a firm body, curly kale will work well in all the recipes that follow. Its leaves have a mild flavor and they crisp up nicely when roasted in the oven, making them ideal for recipes like Roasted Kale Chips (page 42) and Dark Tropical Kiss (page 140).

Lacinato

Lacinato kale (aka dinosaur kale) has deep green, narrow leaves with wrinkled raised bumps that look vaguely reptilian. It's widely available in most grocery stores, and, like curly kale, can be used in almost any recipe that calls for kale. It's the most pungent-tasting of the varieties and has a hint of spiciness that works well with cream sauces and meats. It's delicious paired with the spicy sausage and rich sauce in Linguine with Sausage and Kale (page 91).

Kamome

One of the many types of "flowering" kale, Kamome is an ornamental kale often used to adorn flowerbeds. Kamome comes in several stunning hues, including white, fuchsia, and crimson red hearts with an array of green outer leaves. It tends to taste more like red or green cabbage and pairs well in recipes that include soy or vinegar, such as Kung Pao Chicken with Kale (page 116) and Kale Kiwi Gazpacho (page 36).

Redbor

The deep red leaves of this kale are a true head turner. Redbor is primarily used for ornament in gardens but is just as tasty as the other varieties you'll find at your local grocer. Some farmers say the leaves of this kale get sweeter in late fall, after the first frost. If you can find or grow your own Redbor kale, its dark ruby hue is ideal for the Cherry Kale Campari (page 126).

Red Russian

Red Russian is the peacock of the kale family, with striking red leaf stalks and delicate purple veins that run through its silver green leaves. Sweet, tender, with just a hint of spice, it is ideal for Asian dishes that include ingredients like soy, sesame, and ginger, as well as delicately flavored egg dishes. Try using it in Open Sesame (page 78) or the Cheesy Scrambled Eggs and Kale (page 27).

Love Her Molecules

*T*he father of medicine, Hippocrates, said famously, "Let thy food be thy medicine and medicine be thy food." It seems clear that he was talking about his mistress, kale. To truly know and love kale deeply, you must be intimate with her on a molecular level. The web of atoms she brings together in her unique leaves has the power to heal and soothe you. Here's a brief overview of the attributes she offers.

Folate

The signature B-vitamin of leafy greens, folate derives its name from the Latin word *folium*, which means foliage or leaf. Needed for every cell to replicate and to produce molecules like serotonin that regulate mood, folate is vital for feeling vibrant and vivacious.

ALA

The shortest of the essential omega-3 fats, alpha-linoleic acid (ALA) is fundamental to health. Linked to a variety of benefits like lowering the risk of depression and diabetes, omega-3s are natural soothers. Studies show this fat can help lower anxiety and decrease the effect of stress hormones.

Sulforaphane

One of her most powerful phytonutrients, this sulfur-containing gem is a proven cancer fighter. This molecule naturally ramps up your body's detoxifying enzymes so you zap toxins faster. Regular kale consumption means you are detoxing safely and naturally.

Magnesium

Along with its twin, manganese, magnesium is a key catalyst that drives hundreds of your body's most important chemical reactions. Most people don't get enough magnesium in their diet and some studies have linked low magnesium consumption to an increased risk of diabetes.

Kaempferol

If the fountain of youth exists, it's laced with this powerful molecule. Kaemperfol is one of two molecules shown to extend life by its ability to stimulate the sirtuin genes, also known as the "longevity genes." It is also one of the only molecules known to boost mitochondria, which act as the powerhouses for the cells in our bodies.

Fiber

A healthy gut is key to overall health and well-being. Fiber is an underappreciated nutrient. Large and undigestible, it helps your body excrete cholesterol and bile as it passes through your intestines.

Quercetin

This flavanol antioxidant is key to the health benefits of a plant-based diet. It neutralizes inflammation, protecting the health of your blood vessels, and helps prevent the formation of plaques. It is also a cancer fighter and uses at least three separate mechanisms to help promote the health of your cells.

Iron

Every spark of pleasure and pain requires the explosion of one molecule of oxygen. Iron carries oxygen safely throughout your body. How important is iron? Unlike most vitamins and minerals, you have no way to get rid of iron—your body is built to absorb it. It is a key co-factor for the chemical reactions that make the two brain molecules most related to pleasure: serotonin and dopamine.

Kale Chemistry

While kale is delicious all on her own, she's even more captivating when the chemistry is right. There's nothing strange about these bedfellows from your pantry and fridge—they will make your kale dazzle with robust flavors and unique health synergies. After all, chemistry is everything.

Garlic

"Garlic makes it good," as the old adage says, and new research says that eating garlic on a regular basis can help lower blood pressure. You can add a minced garlic clove to any of the savory garlic dishes or try the Kale Drizzle (page 80) to get your garlicky kale fix.

Ginger

Ginger contains gingerols, which are powerful antibacterial molecules that also can calm nausea and heartburn. Finely grate a few teaspoons of fresh ginger root and toss it with your kale before making Kale Chips (page 42). Or add grated ginger to the pan as you sauté your kale for a little spicy, low-cal zing.

Walnuts and Brazil Nuts

A handful of chopped nuts delivers a pleasant crunch and a rich taste to kale salads as well as to steamed or sautéed kale. Walnuts provide a nice dose of omega-3 fatty acids, while Brazil nuts are high in selenium, a vital mineral needed for healthy hair and metabolism regulation. While nuts offer protein and many health benefits, they are calorie-dense. So if you're watching your waistline, try using a microplane to finely grate nuts over your kale leaves for extra crunch without a lot of added calories.

Caramelized Onions

Deceptively sweet and rich, caramelized onions may taste sinful, but they get their flavor from slow, steady cooking that brings out their natural flavors. To make this luscious topping for kale, heat a large skillet over high heat. Add one tablespoon of olive oil and two thinly sliced onions. Add a pinch of brown sugar and salt. Stir and reduce the heat to medium. Cook 20 to 25 minutes, stirring often until the onions start to soften and brown. If the onions begin to burn or stick, add a few tablespoons of water and continue cooking.

Cocoa

Dark cocoa powder may seem like an unlikely match, but mistress kale knows all about the "dark side." Cocoa and kale make a nice match in smoothies, shakes, and desserts. Just be sure to add a hint of sweetness, such as honey, brown sugar, or stevia to make unsweetened cocoa powder a bit more subtle in your drink.

Exotic Salts

Regular kosher or sea salt brings out kale's flavor, but when you sprinkle on some fancier salts—you really dress her up. Try finishing your kale side dishes and salads with exotic salts, such as pink Himalayan salt, fleur de sel, or smoked sea salt. You can experiment with different flavors without adding extra calories, and provide yourself with the spice of life: variety!

Hot Chilies

Kale can take the heat! Pair cooked kale with pickled jalapeño, canned chipotles, or, if you're very brave, minced habaneros. Spicy chilies can perk up sleepy taste buds while calming an overactive appetite, and may even temporarily increase metabolism.

Lemon

Zesty, refreshing lemon can sweep kale off her feet. Add the juice of one lemon to a raw kale salad or lightly cooked kale, or sprinkle some lemon zest onto any variety of kale dishes, from Kale-slaw (page 50) to Risotto (page 71) for burst of brightness. Adding lemon juice helps your body absorb the iron in kale, and the peel contains two molecules, naringenin and hesperetin, that bind to your opioid receptors and naturally diminish pain while enhancing pleasure.

Parmesan

Kale loves to get a little cheesy—especially with a nice quality Parmesan. The fats in Parmesan can help anchor the antioxidants in kale for better uptake in the body and help you to feel full and satisfied. Finely grated Parmesan delivers a nutty tang that brings out the earthiness in kale, and delivers vital minerals like zinc, magnesium, and B_{12}.

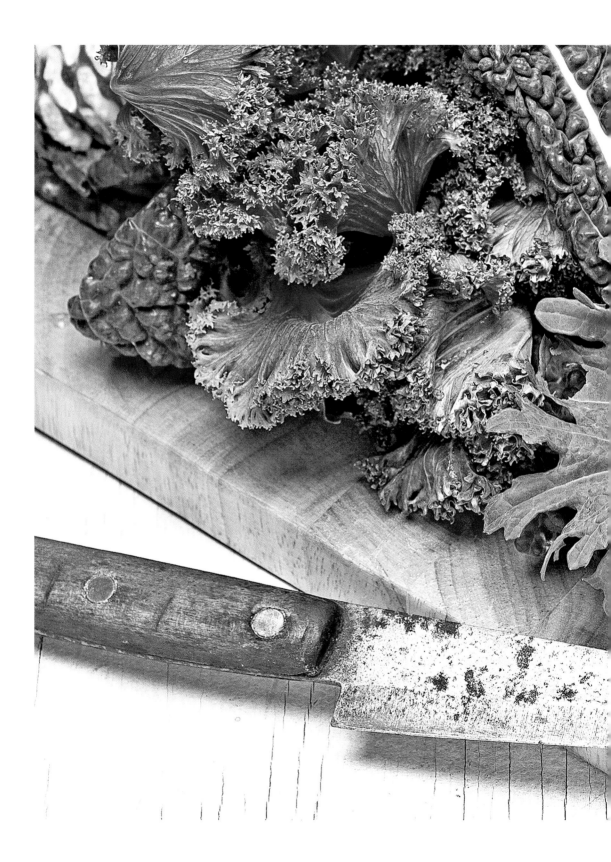

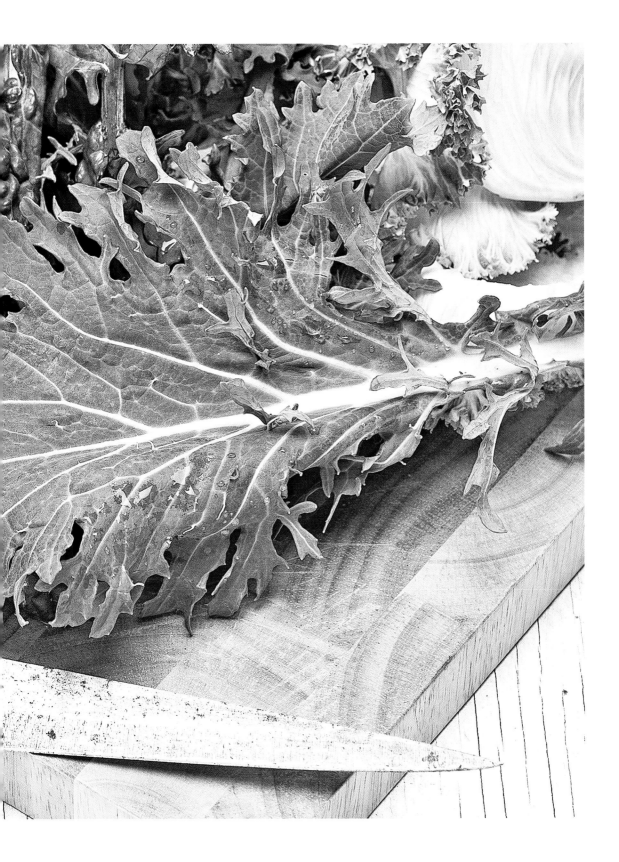

Treat Her Right

Kale is no ordinary vegetable; she offers a seriously impressive list of vitamins and antioxidants that can easily be damaged by overcooking. Here are a few rules of engagement for treating her right.

Steaming

Lightly steaming kale in 1 inch of boiling water ensures that the vitamin C (a water-soluble vitamin) doesn't leach out. Try topping steamed kale with some sliced avocado, fresh-squeezed lemon juice, and a sprinkle of sea salt, or toss with fiber-rich beans for a heartier dish.

Roasting

Roasting kale for a short period of time won't damage nutrients and results in a delightful alternative to traditional snack chips. Just rub your washed, thoroughly dried kale leaves with a little olive oil and sprinkle with your favorite spices. Spread out the seasoned leaves on a baking sheet and roast at 400°F for about 8–10 minutes, or until crispy. Eat as a snack or use as an accompaniment to soups or sandwiches.

Sautéing

Sautéing kale in a healthy fat like olive oil or grapeseed oil is a quick, easy way to create a delicious side dish. Heat a skillet over medium heat and add a tablespoon or two of oil and some chopped kale. Toss and cook for 1 to 2 minutes, until the kale wilts. Top with Parmesan cheese, toasted nuts, or dried fruit for extra flavor.

Raw

Raw kale is delicious in a simple chopped salad. Just stem and chop the kale leaves into bite-sized pieces, then toss with your favorite dressing. Refrigerate for 2 to 3 hours until the kale softens, and enjoy.

Coupling with Kale

When it comes to selecting partners for kale, be picky. Choose the best. She deserves it, and so do you. Here are a few matchmaking pointers. Remember, the quality of ingredients you use affects not only the taste of the recipe, but the health benefits it will offer.

Fruits and Vegetables

Organic produce is always best, but choosing organic does matter more for some fruits and vegetables than others. Conventional peppers, cherries, spinach, blueberries, potatoes, and celery are all more likely to be contaminated with pesticides than their organic counterparts. Always select organic produce in those cases, and be sure to thoroughly wash any produce you buy under warm water before using it. If you're unsure about which fruits and vegetables warrant the extra cost of organic, check out the Environmental Protection Agency (EPA) website for a list of the "Dirty Dozen" and the "Clean Fifteen" at www.ewg.org/foodnews.

Eggs

Whole eggs contain a treasure chest of nutrients, including every essential amino acid the body requires, as well as choline, a compound that promotes memory retention. Whenever possible, select farm-fresh eggs from pasture-raised chickens. They are tastier and healthier, and make you happier, and not just from gazing into your farmer's eyes. The bright yellow yolk in a farm-fresh egg comes from a higher concentration of carotenoids, fat-soluble antioxidants that help to protect your brain. Studies show that these eggs also have higher concentrations of nutrients like vitamin E and omega-3 fats too. If you aren't able to get eggs this close to the source, most grocery stores now carry a wide variety of options. Look for eggs that are labeled "pasture raised," "cage-free," "organic," "vegetarian fed," or "humanely raised." Another option may be to visit your local food cooperative.

Dairy

Tired of skimming the surface? Craving some sweet, rich creaminess in your life? While low-fat milk has become the default choice among health-conscious consumers, you can indulge in the real stuff with a simple shift in the quality of your milk. Just go grass-fed and organic whenever possible. The same rule applies for other dairy products like cheese, sour cream, yogurt, and cream cheese.

Milk-producing cows, sheep, and goats have ruminant stomachs that digest grass and vegetation. When these animals are allowed to graze, they create a special fat called CLA (conjugated linoleic acid), which is linked to a decreased risk of heart disease and diabetes. CLA has even been shown to help fight belly fat. Researchers who have studied populations of people who consume whole-milk, grass-fed dairy products on a regular basis have not been able to identify a clear correlation between full-fat dairy intake and disease in humans.

Dairy has landed on many people's list of foods to avoid mainly due to concerns about lactose intolerance and milk allergies. If you are one of them, the good news is that the majority of recipes in this book are dairy-free or call for small amounts of dairy products. Lactose intolerance can sometimes be managed by cooking with harder, aged cheeses and fermented dairy products like yogurt, or by consuming lactose-free dairy products. Some people who have struggled with

either intolerance or allergies to dairy have reported experiencing fewer symptoms when consuming raw milk or goat's and sheep's milk products. For those of you who simply must avoid dairy, use the dairy imitation products that have worked the best for you.

Meat and Poultry

Meat is so much more than . . . just a piece of meat. While you do want to limit your red meat consumption to a few times per week, this carnal pleasure is well worth the indulgence when you select grass-fed beef. It, too, contains CLA, as well as higher levels of important antioxidants like vitamin E and beta-carotene as compared to conventional beef. Grass-fed beef is also lower in calories—a 6-ounce serving contains about 92 fewer calories than conventional beef.

Luscious, juicy red meat is also an incredibly rich source of heme iron, which has higher absorption rates in the body compared to the non-heme iron found in plants (although when it comes to kale, a unique synergy exists: pairing it with red meat actually *increases* the body's absorption of the iron in kale).

When choosing other red meat products like bacon and sausage, select nitrate-free varieties whenever possible.

Nitrates can be converted into cancer-causing compounds in the stomach. And when it comes to poultry, try to eat pasture-raised birds. Not only will you avoid any concern about the toxins that may be present in conventionally raised birds, but you can't beat the flavor of a bird raised in its natural environment. The best-tasting birds can be bought from your local farmer or farmers' market. Two great online resources for locating local poultry and other locally raised or grown foods in your town are eatwild.com and localharvest.org.

Seafood

We've all been told that seafood is good for our health, but many people remain wary of cooking fresh seafood at home. Two economical, easy-to-prepare, and nutrient-packed choices are wild shrimp and farmed mussels. In general when it comes to fish, it's best to go wild. Farmed fish and shrimp can contain high levels of manmade, environmental toxins. Exposure to these pollutants can lead to impaired brain development, disruption of hormone and immune functions, and increased risk of cancer. In addition, farmed seafood contains lower levels of brain-building omega-3 fats. There is only one exception to this rule: Farmed mussels are generally a great

choice. Not only do they contain high levels of vitamin B$_{12}$, but mussel farms are also safe for the environment, as they act as a filter for the surrounding waters.

Nuts and Seeds

Eating nuts and seeds is a great way to add vital minerals like manganese, magnesium, and zinc into your diet. Studies show that magnesium can promote increased testosterone levels, which is important for sex drive in both men and women. New research suggests that nuts and seeds are a wonder food when it comes to heart health and can drastically cut your chance of coronary heart disease.

Nuts and seeds have a fairly short shelf life of about six months if they are stored unopened in a dark, cool cabinet. If your nuts or seeds have a sharp smell, like paint, chances are they are spoiled. Since nuts and seeds are high in fat, it's best to store them in the fridge instead of a pantry to prevent them from becoming rancid. You can even freeze nuts for up to a year in a well-sealed container.

Toasting nuts and seeds brings out their flavor, and it's so easy to do. Simply place a small, dry skillet over medium-low heat and add the nuts or seeds. Toast for 8 to 10 minutes, stirring often, until they are golden brown and fragrant.

Pantry

*D*o you have the goods? A well-stocked pantry is a sign that you're fully equipped to take your passion for good food to the next level. When you have everything you need on hand, not only are you more likely to spend more time cooking, but you can lose yourself in the act because you don't have to worry about running out to the grocery store to pick up a missing ingredient. Here is a list of some essentials to keep on hand. These basics will help you indulge even your deepest, darkest kale fantasies.

Spices

black peppercorns
Chinese five spice
crushed red pepper flakes
fennel seeds
ground cinnamon
ground coriander
ground cumin
ground nutmeg
sea salt
sesame seeds
sweet or mild chili powder

Oils

canola oil
olive oil
sesame oil

Bottled/jarred

apple cider vinegar
balsamic vinegar
barbecue sauce
honey mustard
jarred salsa, red and green
low-sodium soy sauce
low-sugar orange marmalade
sherry vinegar
Sriracha chili sauce
Worcestershire sauce

Baking

baking powder
baking soda
brown sugar
cacao nibs
cornstarch
granulated white sugar
honey, preferably local
molasses

old-fashioned oats

superfine sugar

sweetened coconut

unsweetened cocoa powder

vanilla extract

white whole wheat flour or
    pastry flour

70% cocoa semisweet chocolate chips

Canned

canned beans: black beans,
    garbanzo beans

canned chipotle chiles

canned tomatoes: whole peeled
    tomatoes, diced tomatoes

low-sodium vegetable broth

tomato paste

Pasta and grains

risotto rice (such as Arborio)

short-grain brown rice

small pasta such as orzo

soba or ramen noodles

taco shells

white or red quinoa

whole grain pastas

whole wheat flour

whole wheat linguine

Nuts and seeds

almonds

pistachios

pumpkin seeds

sesame seeds

walnuts

Now that you've become acquainted with kale—her incredible attributes, her friends and partners, and the best ways to handle her—you're ready to dive into a true love affair. You'll never think of kale as "just a leafy green" again. This romance is not only sustainable, but it's actually healthy—and satisfying. It's time to get a little dirty in the kitchen. Let's dig in. . . .

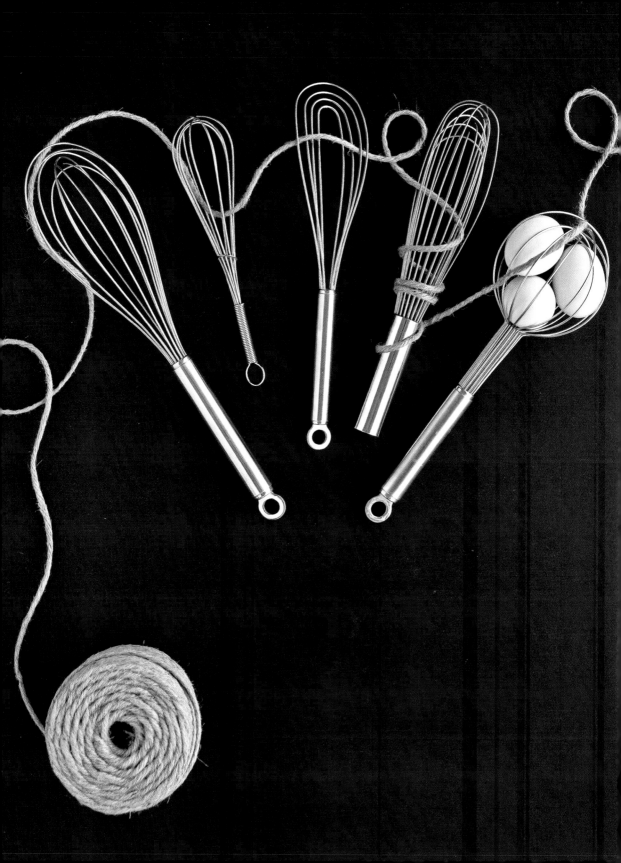

2.

Morning 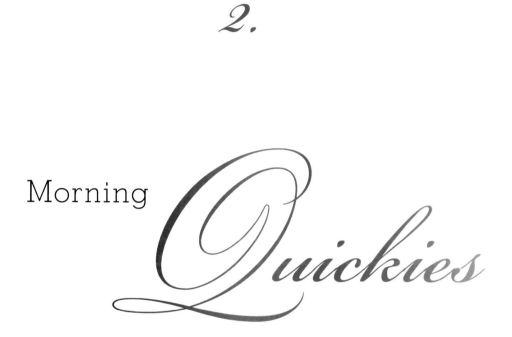 Quickies

Huevos Rancheros

Good morning, cowboy! The traditional breakfast of Latin cowboys, huevos rancheros provided the nutrients they needed for a long day of roping little dogies. With more than 100 percent of your recommended daily needs for vitamin A and 400 percent of your vitamin C requirement, this breakfast offers you the energy you need to fuel your active morning. **Serves 4**

1 tablespoon olive oil

1 red onion, chopped

1 link chorizo, chopped

One 15-ounce can reduced-sodium black beans, well rinsed and drained

½ cup water

5 ounces kale, trimmed and chopped (about 5 cups)

4 eggs

4 small corn tortillas

4 tablespoons jarred salsa

1 jalapeño or other fresh chile, thinly sliced, optional

4 lime wedges, optional

➤ Heat a large skillet over high heat and add the olive oil. Add the onion and chorizo and cook for 3 to 4 minutes, stirring often, until the onion becomes soft and the chorizo is fragrant.

➤ Add the beans and cook for 1 minute more, mashing them with the back of a spoon. Add the water along with the kale, then stir. Cook for about 1 minute more, until half of the liquid evaporates and the kale starts to soften.

➤ Crack the eggs on top of the bean-kale mixture, spacing them an inch apart. Cover and reduce the heat to low. Let the eggs steam for about 1 minute, until the whites are cooked through but the yolks are still soft.

➤ Set out 4 plates and place 1 tortilla on each. Spoon the egg and bean mixture onto the tortillas and top with the salsa. Add the chile and lime, if using, and serve immediately.

PER SERVING (1 EGG, 2 CUPS VEGETABLES, 1 TORTILLA): 305 calories, 16 g protein, 31 g carbohydrates, 14 g fat (4 g saturated), 198 mg cholesterol, 7 g fiber, 508 mg sodium

Did You Know? Beans and eggs offer a double dose of complete protein, which provides the amino acids tryptophan and tyrosine—both of which are needed by the brain to produce feel-good neurotransmitters.

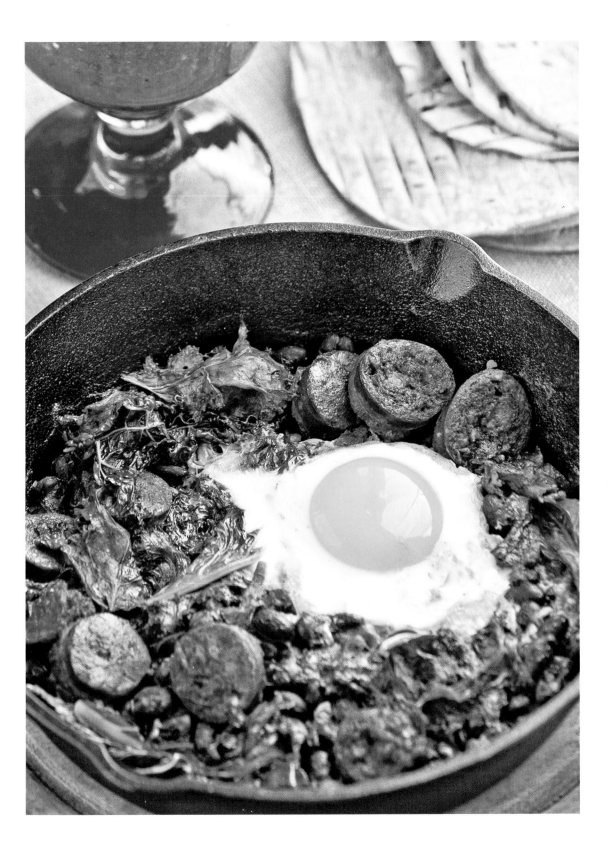

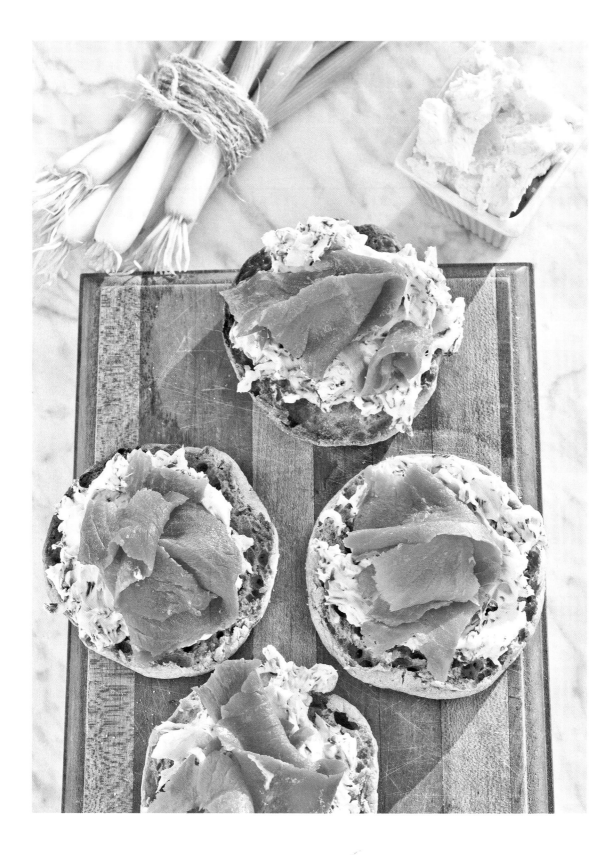

Lox Me Up and Throw Away the Key

Submit to kale in the morning, and feel good all the livelong day. Nestled in cream cheese, scallions and kale combine as a dynamic duo of health-promoting polyphenol antioxidants that fight cancer and promote brain health by reducing inflammation. Anytime is the right time to add more wild salmon into your diet for optimal heart and brain health. It's packed with essential omega-3 fats, which have been shown to fight the blues and stabilize moods. **Serves 4**

1 cup finely chopped kale

1 scallion, thinly sliced

½ cup cream cheese (preferably organic), softened

4 whole wheat English muffins, split and toasted

4 ounces wild smoked salmon, thinly sliced

➤ Place the kale, scallion, and cream cheese in a large bowl. Stir well to combine. Spread the cream cheese over the English muffins. Top each English muffin half with 1 ounce of the smoked salmon, and serve immediately.

PER SERVING (1 ENGLISH MUFFIN WITH TOPPINGS): 267 calories, 14 g protein, 31 g carbohydrates, 12 g fat (5 g saturated), 41 mg cholesterol, 5 g fiber, 595 mg sodium

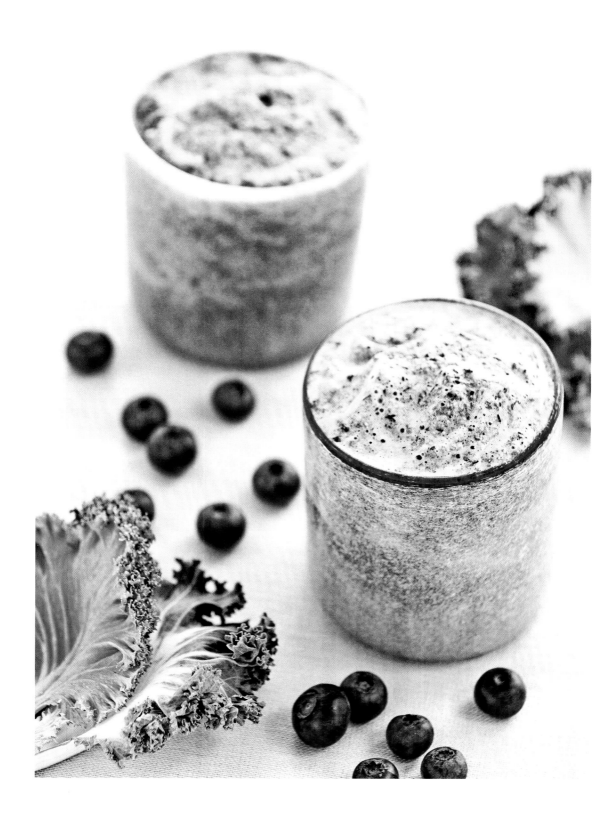

Blueberry Kale Smoothie

This potent smoothie isn't for the weak of heart . . . or then again, maybe it is. It's packed with two key phytonutrients, sulforaphane from kale and anthocyanins from blueberries, both of which are key ingredients for promoting cardiovascular health. They both fight inflammation by eliminating free radicals that, over time, can damage your heart (not to mention your brain, liver, and skin). Like other vegetables, kale offers the most antioxidant value when you eat it raw—so this no-cook smoothie won't lose any nutrition or break your heart. **Serves 1**

1 cup frozen blueberries

½ cup whole milk

½ cup packed roughly chopped kale, stems removed

1 tablespoon honey or agave nectar

½ teaspoon vanilla extract

4 ice cubes

➤ Place all the ingredients in a blender and blend until smooth. Serve immediately.

PER SERVING (2½ CUPS): 243 calories, 6 g protein, 47 g carbohydrates, 4 g fat (2 g saturated), 12 mg cholesterol, 4 g fiber, 69 mg sodium

Did You Know? Organic blueberries offer even more antioxidant value than conventional blueberries. Freezing fresh blueberries when they're in season is a great way to preserve their nutrient value.

Cheddar Kale Omelet

The gooey, melted cheese and golden onions in this omelet are guaranteed to induce lust, but it's the mushrooms that will really bring you to your knees. Their over-the-top richness comes from nineteen amino acids, the fundamental building blocks of cells. A serving of mushrooms also contains 24 percent of your recommended daily allowance (RDA) of niacin, an essential B vitamin needed to produce energy and sex hormones. **Serves 4**

2 tablespoons olive oil

10 ounces mushrooms, such as cremini or white button, sliced

1 sweet white onion, such as Vidalia, sliced

¼ teaspoon salt

5 ounces kale, trimmed and thinly sliced (about 5 cups)

4 eggs

2 slices sharp white cheddar cheese (about 1 ounce)

➤ Heat a large skillet over medium heat. Add 1 tablespoon of the olive oil, the mushrooms, onion, and salt. Cook for 5 to 6 minutes, stirring often, until the mushrooms release their liquid and the volume shrinks by half. Add the kale and cook for 1 to 2 minutes more, pressing down the kale with a small metal lid as you turn it. Turn the heat off and set aside.

➤ Place the eggs in a medium bowl and whisk well. Heat another large skillet over high heat. Pull the skillet off the burner and coat with the remaining 1 tablespoon olive oil, then return it to the heat. Turn the heat down to medium and add the egg mixture. Pull the cooked edges of the eggs back toward the center of the pan and tilt the pan to allow some of the uncooked mixture to settle around the edges. Repeat 2 or 3 times, until you have a thicker center and the egg is almost cooked through.

➤ Spoon the mushroom-kale mixture over half the egg and top with the cheese slices. Cover and cook over low heat for about 1 minute. Flip the edge of the omelet over to form a half moon. Cover to allow the cheese to melt, 25 to 30 seconds. Cut into 4 wedges and serve immediately.

PER SERVING (1 SLICE OMELET, ABOUT 1½ CUPS): 201 calories, 14 g protein, 9 g carbohydrates, 12 g fat (4 g saturated), 201 mg cholesterol, 2 g fiber, 349 mg sodium

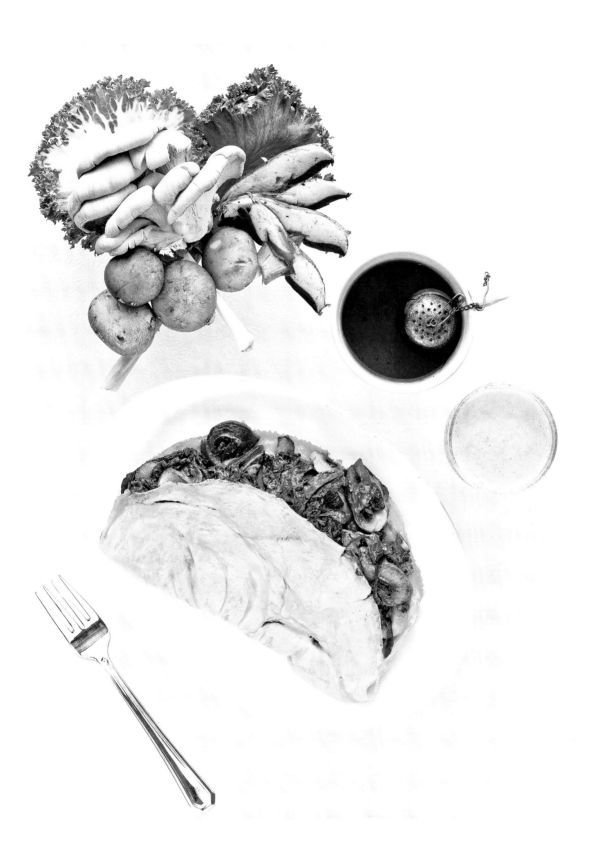

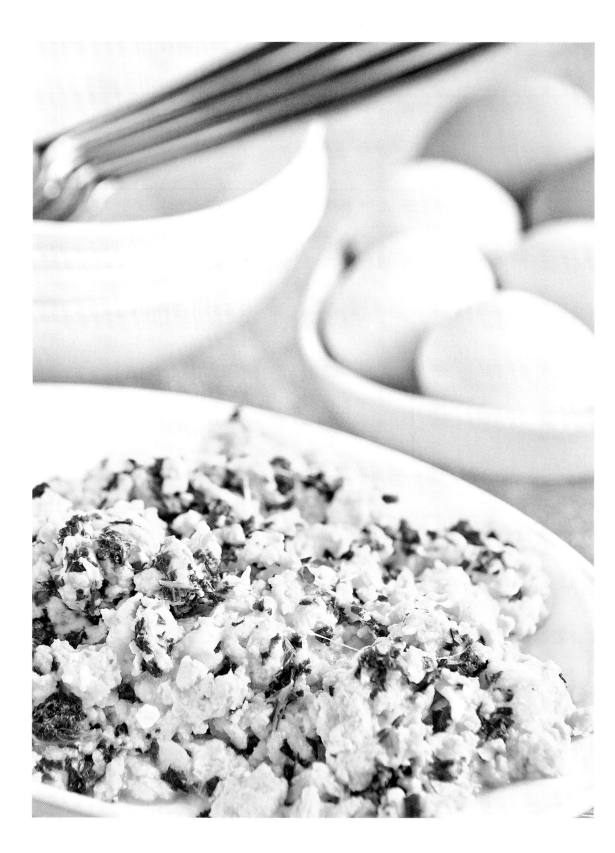

Cheesy Scrambled Eggs and Kale

Scrambled eggs are the ideal "quickie"—they take just minutes to cook. And when you couple kale with eggs, you get a lot of hot love for your body, with all of the essential amino acids, more than forty different flavonoids that help fight aging, and a bangin' amount of vitamins. **Serves 4**

6 eggs

1 tablespoon olive oil

5 ounces kale, trimmed and thinly sliced (about 5 cups)

Olive oil cooking spray

1 cup grated mozzarella or Colby cheese

➤ Place the eggs in a medium bowl and whisk well. Set aside.

➤ Heat a large skillet over medium heat. Add the olive oil and kale and cook for 2 to 3 minutes, pressing down on the kale with a metal lid, turning often until it's soft.

➤ Transfer the kale to a plate. Warm the same skillet (that you cooked the kale in) over medium-high heat. Coat with a thin layer of cooking spray. Add the eggs and cook for 2 to 3 minutes, stirring often, until soft curds form. Add the kale and the cheese and remove from heat. Cover and rest for 1 minute, until the cheese melts. Serve immediately.

PER SERVING (ABOUT 2 CUPS): 252 calories, 18 g protein, 7 g carbohydrates, 17 g fat (6 g saturated), 294 mg cholesterol, 1.5 g fiber, 319 mg sodium

Did You Know? There's no need to stress about the cholesterol in eggs. Most cholesterol in food isn't even absorbed into your body, and there's no conclusive science that links *dietary* cholesterol to your risk of heart disease or stroke. Studies show that up to 7 eggs a week won't affect your blood cholesterol levels.

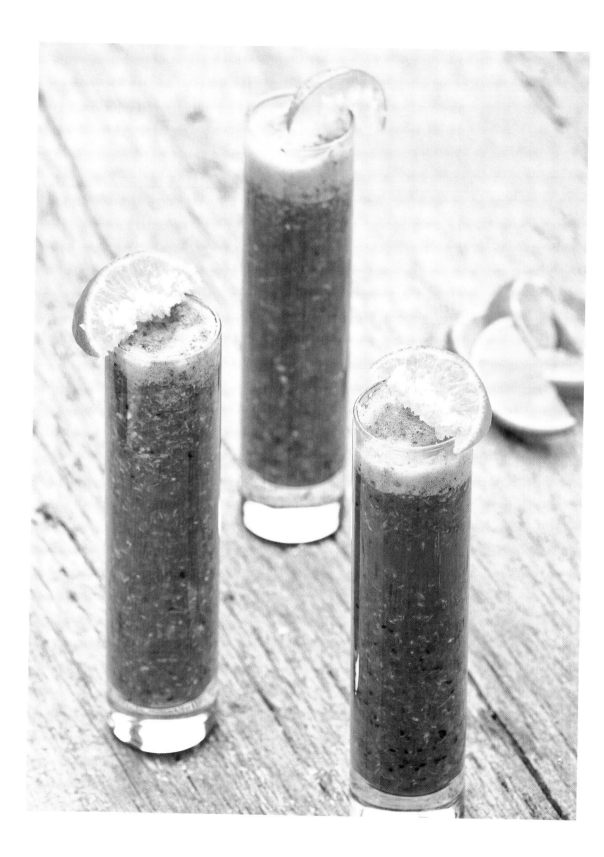

Energy Jolt

Looking to electrify your body and jolt your libido into action? Sip on this smoothie and you'll get 400 percent of your recommended daily need of vitamin C, important for good circulation and blood flow. You'll also get a healthy dose of vitamin A, which helps your body regulate the synthesis of sex hormones all day long. Add some sea salt and lime wedges for a virgin experience that feels a little naughty.

Serves 4

4 cups chopped kale

1 small kiwi, peeled and roughly chopped

One 1-inch piece ginger, peeled and chopped

4 lime wedges dipped into ¼ teaspoon sea salt, optional

➤ Place the kale, kiwi, and ginger in a blender and blend until smooth. Pour into glasses and serve immediately with salt-dipped lime wedges, if using.

PER SERVING (1½ CUPS): 185 calories, 9 g protein, 39 g carbohydrates, 2 g fat (0 g saturated), 0 mg cholesterol, 7 g fiber, 118 mg sodium

Did You Know? Bring on the toys! If you're a die-hard smoothie maker, invest in some serious machinery like the Vitamix or Blendtec blenders. These professional-grade blenders transform the texture of veggies in seconds, from rough and raw to velvety smooth. They're also great for whipping up healthy soups in minutes.

Sunny Side Up with Greens

In this simple but filling breakfast, a luscious egg yolk oozes over kale. Eggs are one of the few foods that provide all of the basic building blocks needed for a healthy, happy, sunny-side-up mood, namely B vitamins folate and B_{12}. Eggs are also the top dietary source of choline, which is linked to lower rates of anxiety—but only if you enjoy the yolk, where these nutrients reside. **Serves 1**

Olive oil cooking spray

3 cups chopped kale

1 egg

⅛ teaspoon salt

1 tablespoon Kale-onaise (page 53) or jarred salsa

2 slices whole wheat or whole grain bread, toasted

➤ Heat a large skillet over high heat. Pull it off the heat and coat with cooking spray. Return it to the heat and carefully add the kale. Cook for 2 to 3 minutes, pressing down the kale with a spatula. Move the kale to the side and add cooking spray to the center of the skillet.

➤ Crack the egg into the center of the skillet and sprinkle it with the salt. Reduce the heat to medium and continue to cook for 3 to 4 minutes, until the white of the egg is cooked through. Top with Kale-onaise or salsa and serve immediately, with the toast.

PER SERVING (1½ CUPS WITH SALSA WITH 2 PIECES OF TOAST): 333 calories, 19 g protein, 48 g carbohydrates, 8 g fat (2 g saturated), 186 mg cholesterol, 8 g fiber, 859 mg sodium

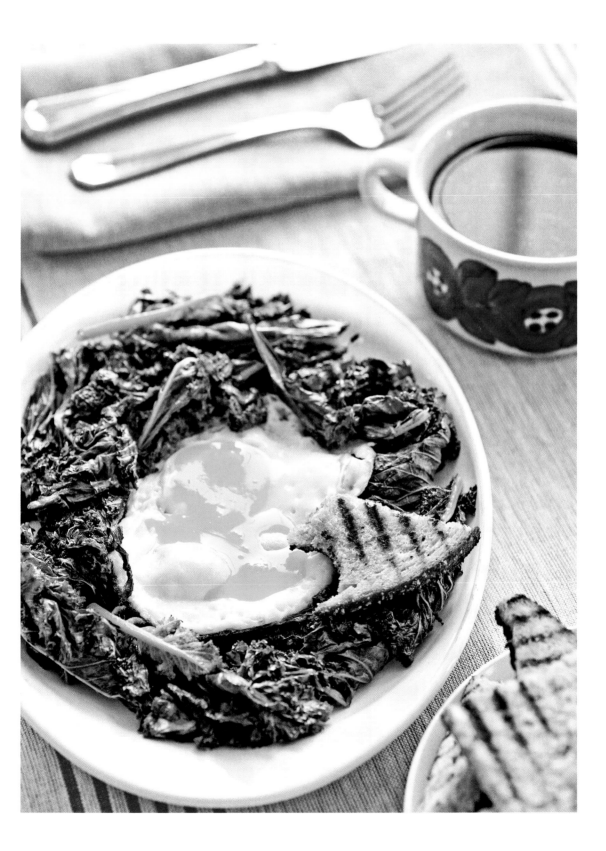

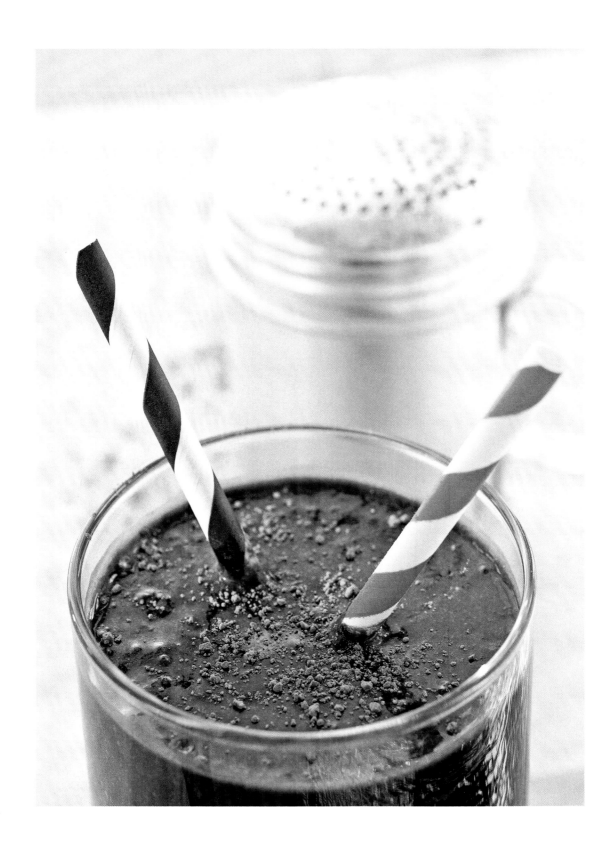

Cocoa Delight

If you have a fetish for dark chocolate, this will fuel your flame. It will also energize your body with antioxidants that boost blood flow to the brain (and a few other vital organs). Cocoa, kale, and cherries, three beloved and sexy superfoods, contain flavonoids and antioxidants that fight heart disease and diabetes and even promote brain growth. **Serves 1**

1 cup roughly chopped kale

1 cup frozen pitted black cherries

2 tablespoons unsweetened cocoa powder, plus 1 teaspoon for sprinkling

2 tablespoons granulated sugar

➤ Place all the ingredients in a blender and blend until smooth. Pour into a glass and sprinkle with the cocoa powder. Serve immediately.

PER SERVING (1 CUP): 151 calories, 4 g protein, 35 g carbohydrates, 1 g fat (0 g saturated), 0 mg cholesterol, 0 g fiber, 29 mg sodium

Did You Know? Chocolate feels naughty but can be nice for your health, as long as you choose a variety that contains 70% cocoa or more. Studies show that the flavonoid antioxidants in chocolate can improve mood, increase blood flow to the brain, and even help lower risk of stroke. Dark chocolate is also an excellent source of minerals such as iron, magnesium, copper, and zinc.

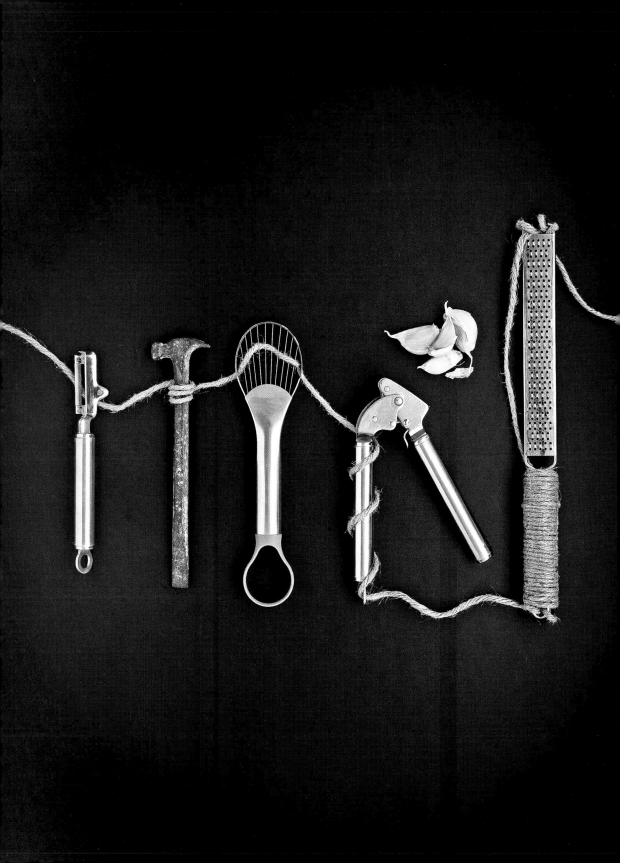

Small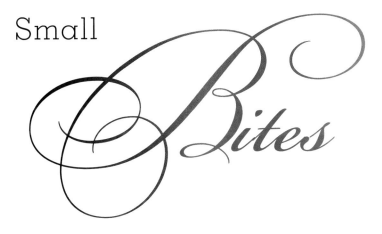

Kale Kiwi Gazpacho

This light and tangy gazpacho makes for a refreshing poolside treat—and at just 110 calories per serving, it also helps you get bikini-ready. Want to really turn up the heat? If you're a chile-lovin' sadist, add the jalapeño seeds to the food processor. Speaking of seeds—those little black kiwi seeds are a great source of ALA omega-3 fats, which are linked to staying young and flexible. Grrrr. **Serves 4**

5 ounces kale, stemmed and chopped (about 5 cups)

2 kiwis, peeled and quartered

1 green bell pepper, cored, seeded, and roughly chopped

1 small jalapeño, quartered and seeded

2 cloves garlic, cut in half

2 tablespoons extra virgin olive oil

2 tablespoons sherry vinegar

½ teaspoon sea salt

➤ Place all the ingredients in a food processor and process until smooth. Cover and chill for 1 hour before serving.

PER SERVING (1 CUP): 110 calories, 2 g protein, 11 g carbohydrates, 7 g fat (1 g saturated), 0 mg cholesterol, 2 g fiber, 213 mg sodium

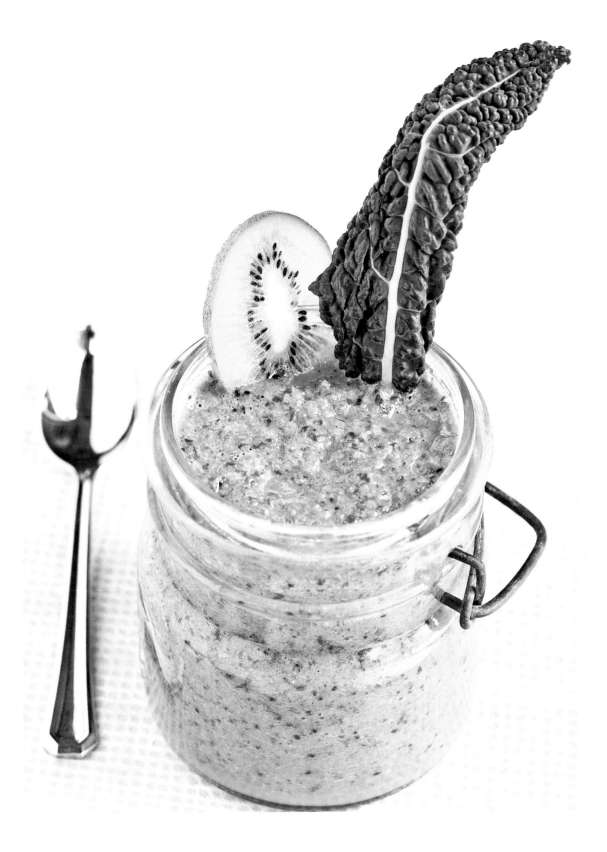

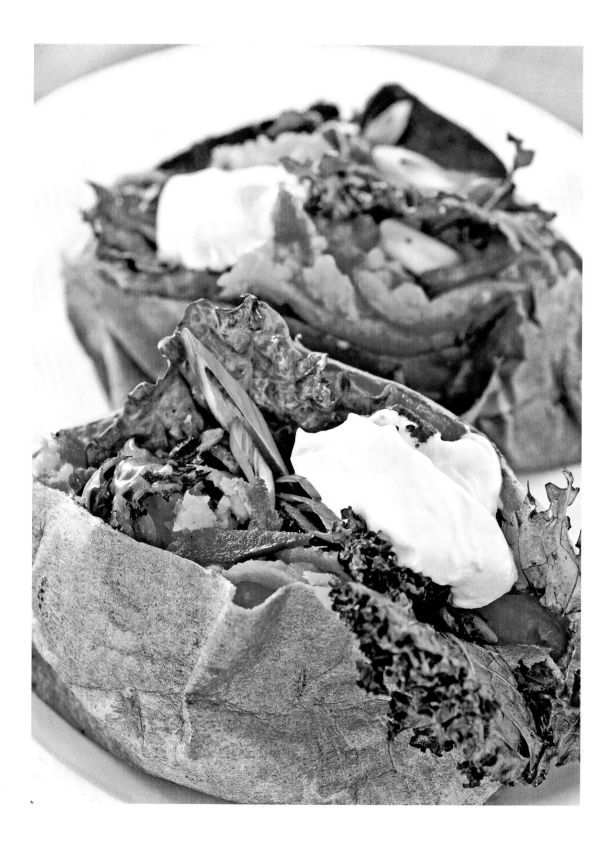

Baked Sweet Potatoes with Kale and Bacon

Sustained passion requires a strong heart and a sexy body. This fiber-rich dish will help to protect your heart *and* keep you trim, since fiber ensures you feel full and satisfied and also helps regulate your blood sugar. Sweet potatoes are also a top source of powerful carotenoid antioxidants, which your body converts to vitamin A—necessary for the health of the organ of seduction: the eyes. **Serves 4**

4 cups chopped kale

1 tablespoon olive oil

4 medium-sized sweet potatoes

4 slices nitrate-free bacon, cooked and crumbled

4 tablespoons sour cream (organic if possible)

4 scallions, thinly sliced

➤ Preheat the oven to 350°F.

➤ Place the kale in a large bowl along with the olive oil. Toss well, coating the leaves, then transfer to an ungreased baking sheet. Poke the sweet potatoes with the tines of a fork and place them on a baking sheet covered with aluminum foil. Bake the sweet potatoes for 1 hour, or until they are soft to the touch. During the last 5 minutes of baking, place kale in the oven.

➤ Make a slit in the top of each sweet potato and transfer them to a plate. Press the sweet potatoes open and top each with a quarter of the baked kale. Next, top each with one quarter of the crumbled bacon, 1 tablespoon of the sour cream, and a quarter of the scallions. Serve immediately.

PER SERVING (1 BAKED SWEET POTATO WITH TOPPINGS): 360 calories, 9 g protein, 65 g carbohydrates, 8 g fat (2 g saturated), 13 mg cholesterol, 10 g fiber, 331 mg sodium

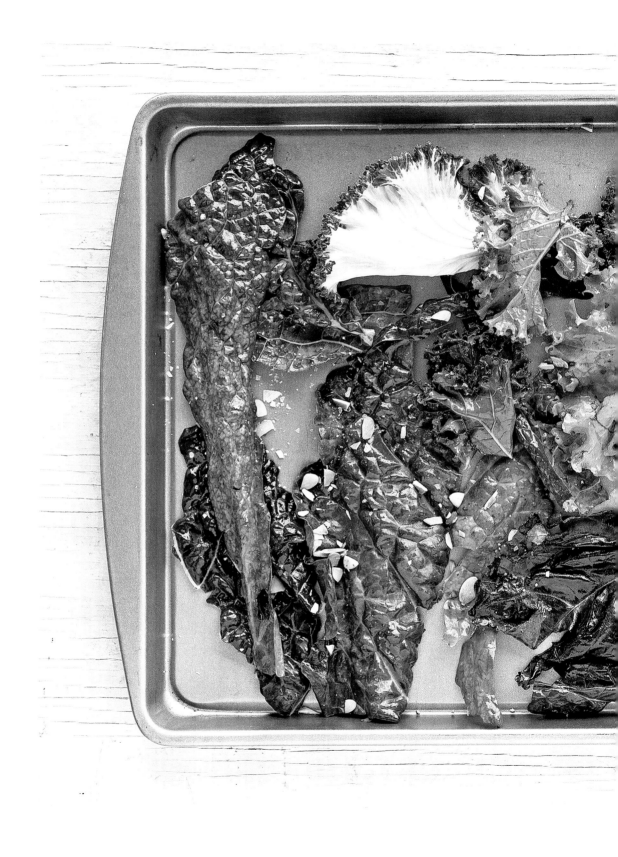

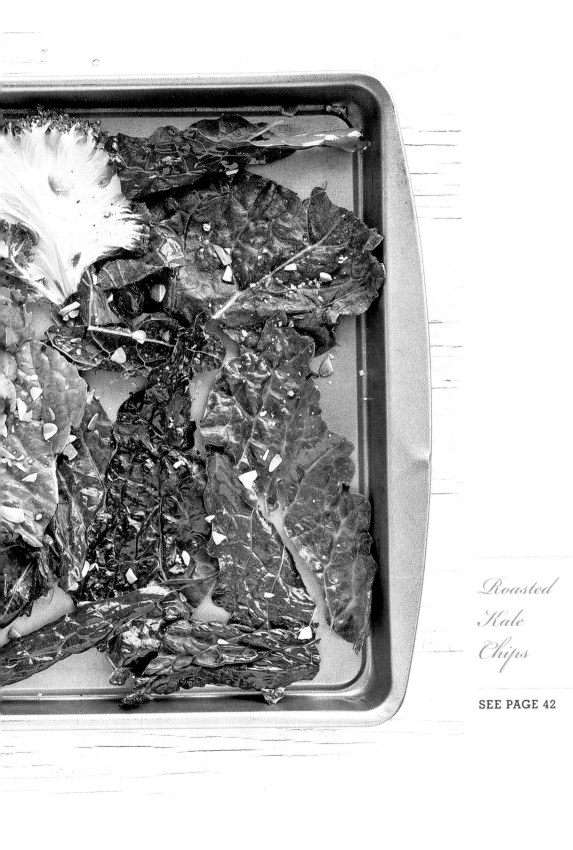

Roasted
Kale
Chips

SEE PAGE 42

Roasted Kale Chips

Snack time—the decision is yours: Do you want to be bad, to feel the weight of your carnal sin all afternoon? Or do you want to indulge your cravings without feeling ashamed? These homemade kale chips have a delicate crunch that makes for a satisfying snack you don't have to feel guilty about. **Serves 4**

One 1½-pound bunch kale

1 tablespoon olive oil

1 tablespoon pumpkin seeds

¼ teaspoon sea salt

¼ teaspoon freshly ground black pepper

➤ Preheat the oven to 350°F and set out 2 ungreased baking sheets with sides.

➤ Rinse the kale under cold running water and pat dry with paper towels. Wrap the kale in another layer of fresh paper towel—the kale must be dry in order to crisp up. Squeeze and unroll.

➤ Roughly chop the kale leaves and discard the stems or reserve them for Simple Chicken Broth (page 108).

➤ In a large bowl, toss the kale leaves with the olive oil, pumpkin seeds, salt, and pepper, rubbing the leaves with your fingers to coat with the oil and spices. Arrange the leaves over the baking sheets and bake for 7 to 8 minutes. If the chips are crisp in the center, remove them from the oven and serve. Otherwise, bake for an additional 2 to 5 minutes, until the chips have crisped.

PER SERVING (2 CUPS): 126 calories, 17 g protein, 17 g carbohydrates, 5 g fat (0.8 g saturated), 0 mg cholesterol, 3 g fiber, 240 mg sodium

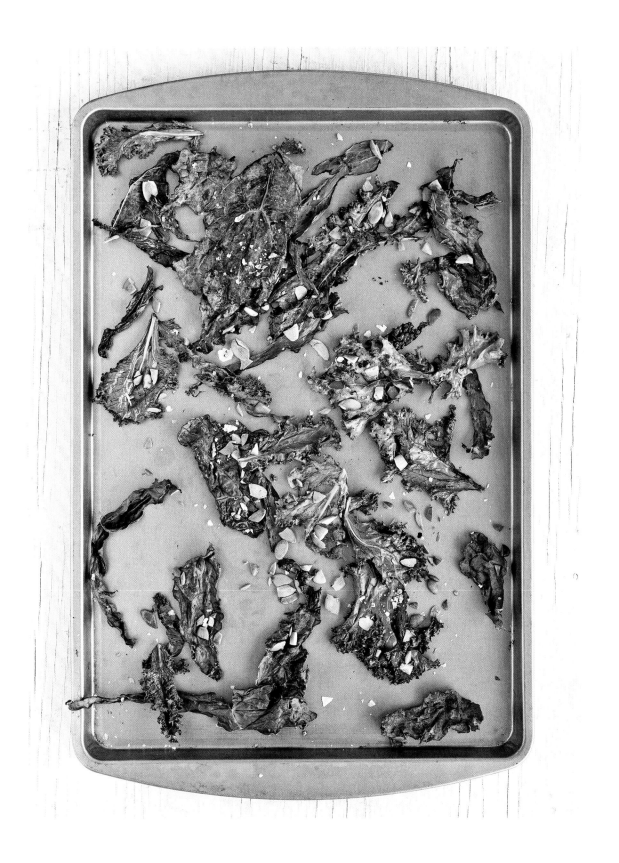

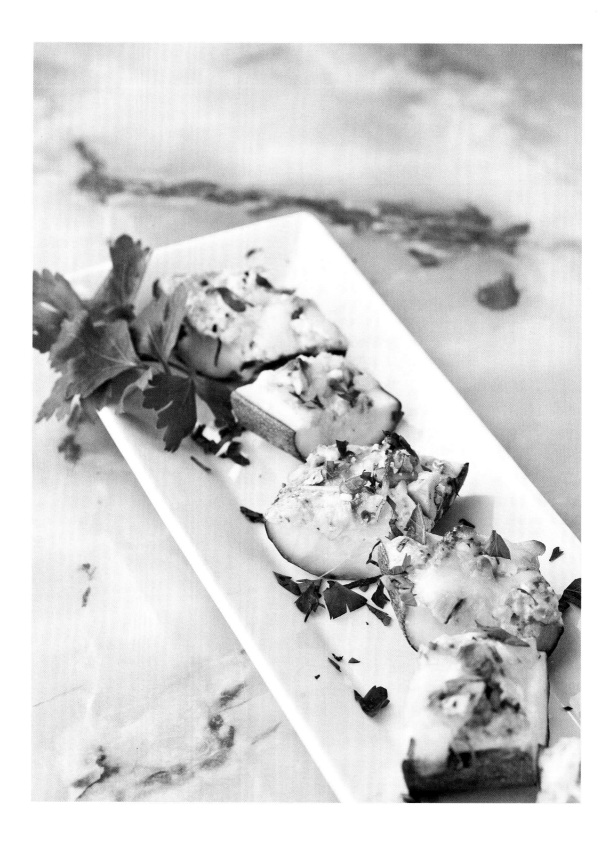

Zucchini and Kale Bites

Serve these elegant canapés as your sweetie walks through the door after work and you're sure to set the mood for the evening to come. You'll also be giving your honey some serious brain food. Walnuts are rich in mood-boosting and nerve-calming omega-3s. **Serves 4**

2 cups roughly chopped kale

½ cup toasted chopped walnuts

2 medium zucchinis, tops removed and cut in half lengthwise

4 tablespoons Kale-onaise (page 53)

1 cup grated Manchego or Parmesan cheese

2 tablespoons minced fresh parsley

Olive oil for drizzling, optional

➤ Preheat the oven to 400°F.

➤ Combine the kale and walnuts in a food processor and process until smooth.

➤ In a large saucepan, steam the zucchini for 8 to 10 minutes, until it begins to soften but is still firm to the touch. Remove and place the zucchini cut side up on a cookie sheet lined with parchment paper or aluminum foil.

➤ In a medium bowl, mix the Kale-onaise, half of the kale mixture, half of the cheese, and 1 tablespoon of the parsley. Cover each half of zucchini with a thin layer of the mixture and top with the remaining cheese.

➤ Drizzle lightly with olive oil, if using, and bake for 20 to 25 minutes, until the cheese bubbles and starts to brown. Allow the zucchini boats to cool for a few minutes, then slice into 2-inch chunks and sprinkle with remaining kale mixture and parsley. Serve warm or at room temperature.

PER SERVING (ABOUT 1 CUP): 243 calories, 10 g protein, 9 g carbohydrates, 19 g fat (5 g saturated), 22 mg cholesterol, 2 g fiber, 244 mg sodium

Hot Bacon Kale and Eggs

Your forbidden pleasure. Bacon. Release yourself from the shame! Bacon offers a healthy dose of thiamine—the B vitamin required for all energy-producing reactions in the body. And you never know when you may end up needing an extra burst of energy. . . . **Serves 4**

4 eggs

8 slices nitrate-free bacon, chopped

One 10-ounce bunch kale, trimmed and chopped (about 10 cups)

¼ cup apple cider vinegar

4 teaspoons granulated sugar

¼ cup water

½ medium red onion, thinly sliced (about ½ cup)

➤ Place the eggs in a small saucepan and cover with cold water. Place over high heat and bring to a boil. Cover and turn off the heat. Leave for 15 minutes. Drain and run the eggs under cold running water. Peel the eggs, chop or quarter them, and set aside.

➤ In a large skillet over medium heat, cook the bacon for 2 to 3 minutes, stirring often, until it is crisp. Transfer it to a large bowl. Turn the heat to medium and add the kale. Cook for 2 to 3 minutes, pressing it down with a small metal lid to wilt it. Carefully add the vinegar, sugar, and ¼ cup water. Using a wooden spoon, scrape up any bits of bacon sticking to the bottom of the pan. Transfer the kale along with any sauce remaining in the skillet to a platter. Top with the egg and onion and serve immediately.

PER SERVING (2½ CUPS): 204 calories, 15 g protein, 9 g carbohydrates, 12 g fat (4 g saturated), 204 mg cholesterol, 1 g fiber, 472 mg sodium

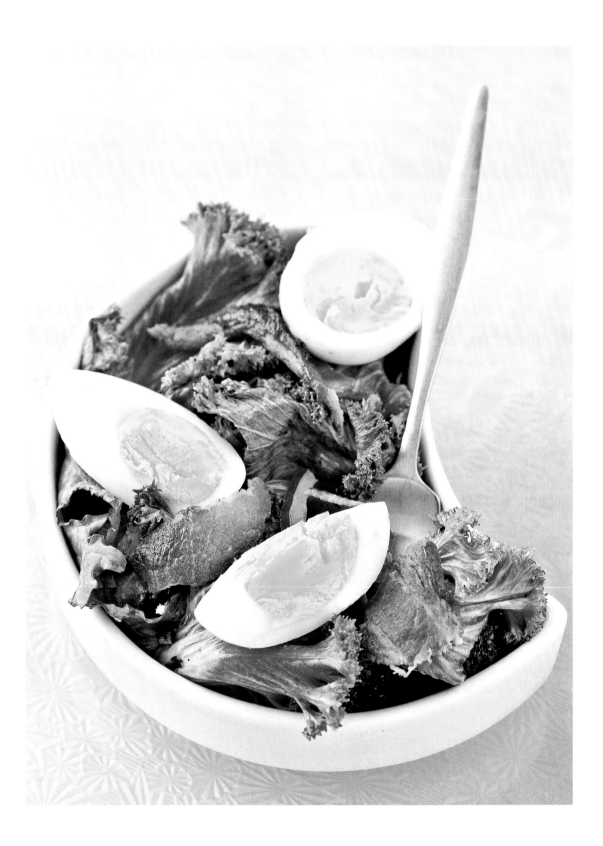

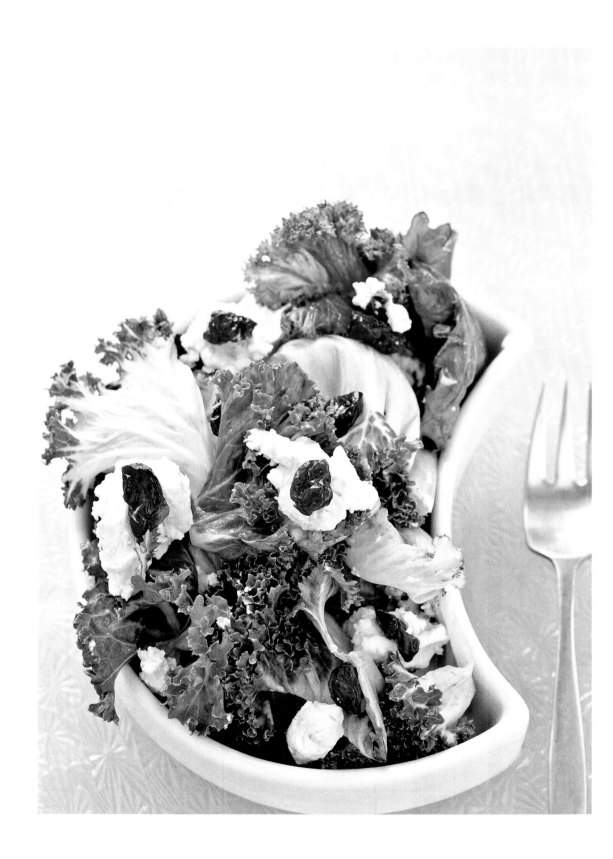

Kale with Goat Cheese and Dried Cherries

Looking for some love on the side? If you're a kale newbie, this is a great place to start. Tangy dried cherries and velvety goat cheese make it hard to resist falling for this sweet and savory salad. **Serves 4**

1 tablespoon olive oil

One 10-ounce bunch kale, trimmed and chopped (about 10 cups)

½ teaspoon sea salt

½ cup dried cherries

2 ounces soft goat cheese, cut into ½-inch cubes

➤ Heat a large skillet over high heat. Add the olive oil, kale, and salt. Cook for 2 to 3 minutes, pressing down the kale with a small metal lid, and turning often. Add the cherries and goat cheese and cover to allow the cheese to melt. Transfer to a large platter and serve immediately.

PER SERVING (1 CUP): 153 calories, 5 g protein, 22 g carbohydrates, 7 g fat (2 g saturated), 6 mg cholesterol, 2 g fiber, 85 mg sodium

Kaleslaw

You may not think of coleslaw as sexy, and you'd be right—most coleslaw is far from a turn-on. But this colorful, lighter version brings the sexy back with superfoods carrots and red, yellow, or orange bell peppers. It's also a great way to enjoy your kale in the raw. **Serves 8**

One 10-ounce bunch kale, stemmed and roughly chopped (about 10 cups)

6 carrots

1 red, yellow, or orange bell pepper, cored, seeded, and diced or thinly sliced

1½ cups Kale-onaise (page 53)

➤ Fit a food processor with the shredder attachment. Shred the kale and carrots and transfer both to a large bowl. Add the bell pepper and Kale-onaise and toss well. Cover and refrigerate for at least 1 hour or up to overnight before serving.

PER SERVING (1 CUP): 187 calories, 3 g protein, 10 g carbohydrates, 16 g fat (2 g saturated), 8 mg cholesterol, 2 g fiber, 591 mg sodium

Did You Know? When it comes to health, mayo gets a bad rap because it's often a highly processed food. But both traditional mayonnaise and modern canola oil–based versions are healthy in moderation. Most mayonnaise contains monounsaturated and polyunsaturated fats, two fats that are actually good for you.

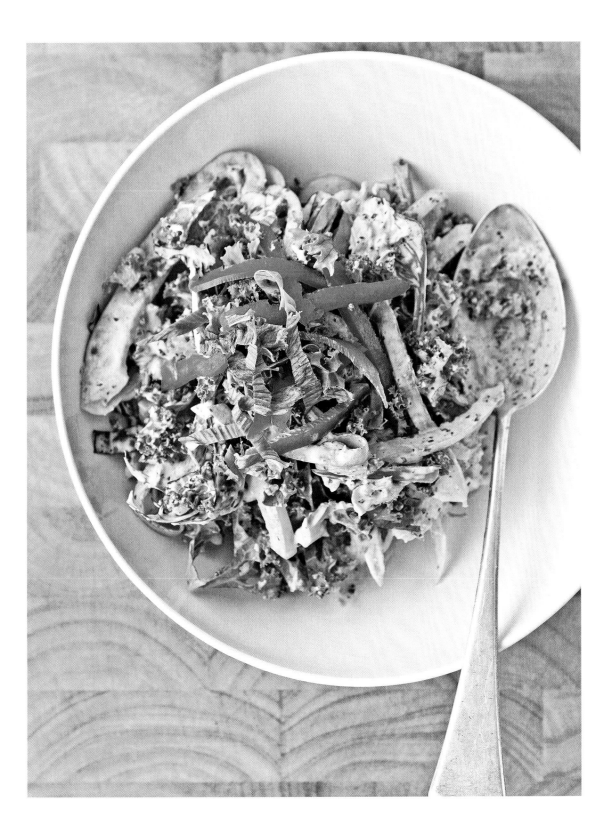

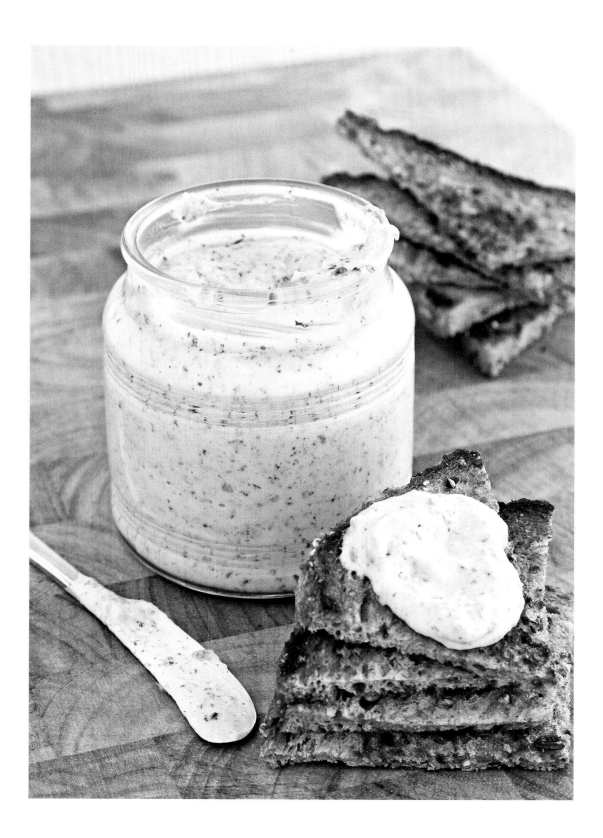

Kale-onaise

Dress up any dip, sandwich, or dressing with this flavorful and healthy mayo that also offers the nutrient value of raw kale and fresh garlic. This creamy condiment will soon take the place of butter on your breakfast toast. Go ahead, we won't watch. Spread 'em. **Makes 3 cups**

2 cups packed chopped kale

½ teaspoon sea salt

2 garlic cloves, chopped

1 cup mayonnaise (organic if possible)

Zest and juice of 1 lemon

➤ In a food processor, combine the kale leaves, salt, and garlic. Process until finely chopped. Add the mayonnaise and lemon zest and juice and process until smooth.

PER SERVING (2 TABLESPOONS): 60 calories, 0 g protein, 0 g carbohydrates, 7 g fat (1 g saturated), 3 mg cholesterol, 0 g fiber, 93 mg sodium

Did You Know? Fresh garlic, like kale, contains sulfur compounds that become more available to your body after crushing it or mixing it with lemon juice. Garlic has been shown to help protect the heart and the brain by lowering inflammation in blood vessels.

Goddess Guacamole

This rich guacamole is the ideal skinny dip. Creamy avocado isn't just velvety-smooth on the tongue—it also helps to keep your skin soft and supple thanks to its pro-vitamin A compounds, which are thought to help prevent wrinkles. **Serves 4**

2 cups torn kale leaves

4 ripe Hass avocados

½ teaspoon sea salt, or more to taste

3 ripe tomatoes, seeded and chopped

¼ cup minced red onion

2 jalapeño chiles, seeded and finely chopped

Juice of 1 lime

¼ cup minced fresh cilantro

➤ Place the kale leaves in a food processor and pulse until they are finely chopped. Cut the avocados in half and remove the pits. Scoop out the flesh and place it in a large wooden or metal bowl. Add the salt and mash with the back of a wooden spoon until desired texture is reached—I like mine a bit chunky. Stir in the kale leaves and the remaining ingredients. Taste and adjust the seasonings with salt. Serve immediately, or place a piece of plastic wrap directly over the surface of the dip and store in the refrigerator for up to 10 hours. Serve with whole grain tortilla chips, toasted whole wheat pita wedges, or toasted soft corn tortillas.

PER SERVING (1 CUP): 77 calories, 2 g protein, 8 g carbohydrates, 5 g fat (1 g saturated), 0 mg cholesterol, 4 g fiber, 200 mg sodium

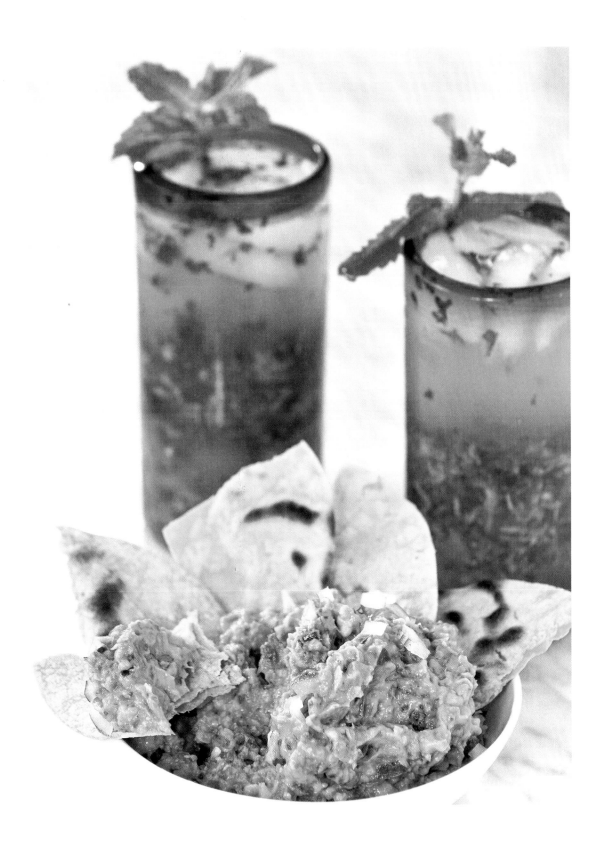

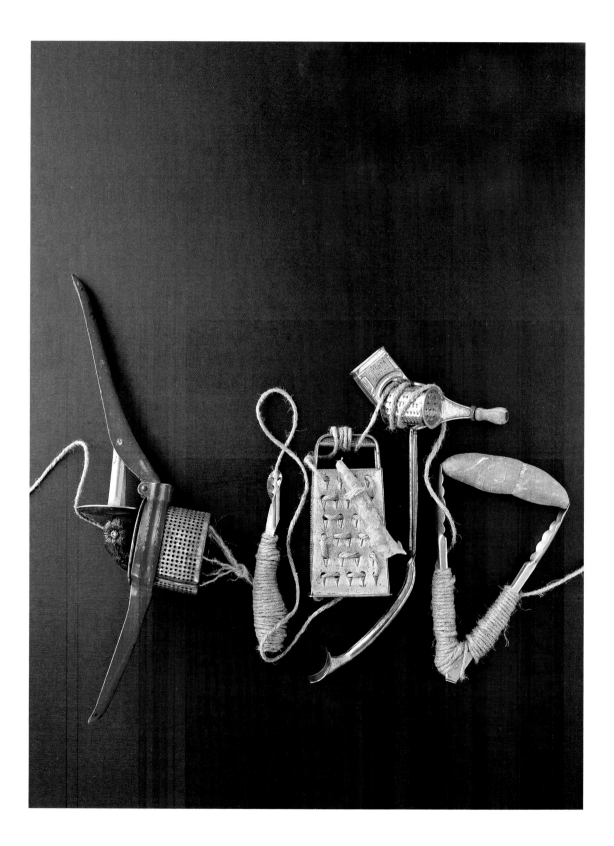

4.

Vegetarian

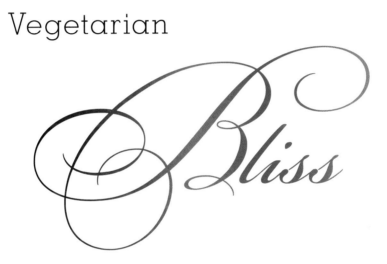
Bliss

Grilled Cheese 'n Kale

No one forgets a childhood love. This classic comfort food makes you feel warm and fuzzy all over . . . and now you can indulge your nostalgia without the guilt. Swapping in whole wheat bread for white and adding a heaping measure of kale ensures that you'll stay fuller longer, since the extra fiber slows digestion and nutrient uptake. Give in and go with the grain . . . it's okay to be a traditionalist sometimes. **Serves 4**

4 tablespoons honey mustard

8 thin slices whole wheat bread

4 ounces mozzarella cheese, grated

Olive oil cooking spray

4 tablespoons unsalted butter

2 cups torn kale leaves

➤ Spread 1 tablespoon of the honey mustard on 4 slices of bread, then sprinkle on the cheese, add the torn kale leaves, and assemble the sandwiches with the remaining 4 slices.

➤ Coat a large skillet with cooking spray and warm it over medium heat. Add 2 tablespoons of the butter. When the butter is melted, transfer the sandwiches to the skillet and cook for 2 to 4 minutes on one side until golden. Spread the top of the sandwiches with the remaining 2 tablespoons of butter and flip. Cook for an additional 2 to 4 minutes, until the cheese is melted. Transfer the sandwiches to a cutting board and cut each in half or into quarters. Serve immediately.

PER SERVING (1 SANDWICH): 390 calories, 16 g protein, 40 g carbohydrates, 18 g fat (10 g saturated), 49 mg cholesterol, 7 g fiber, 591 mg sodium

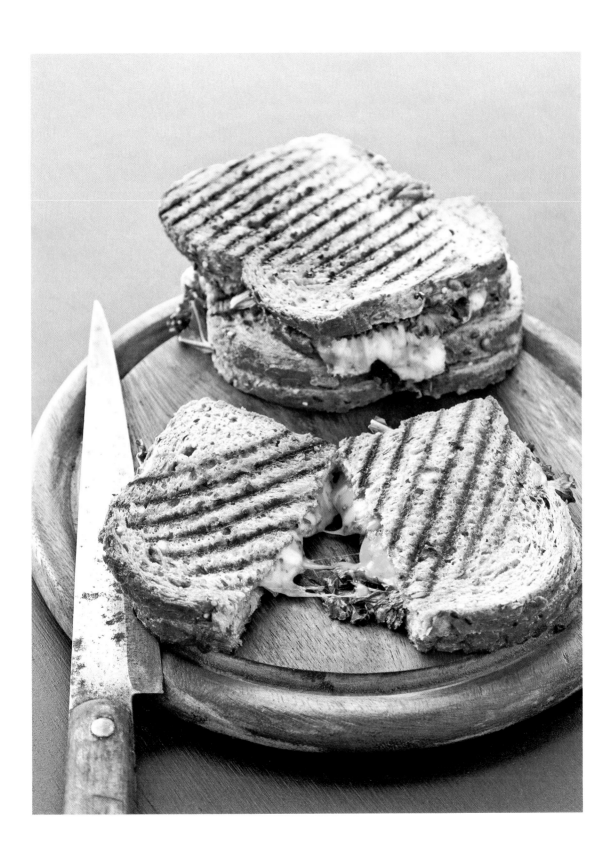

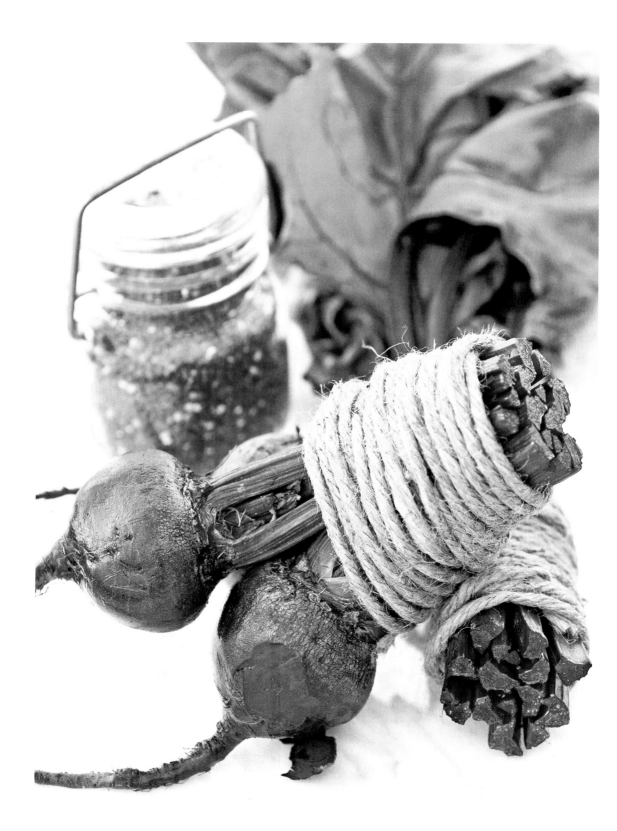

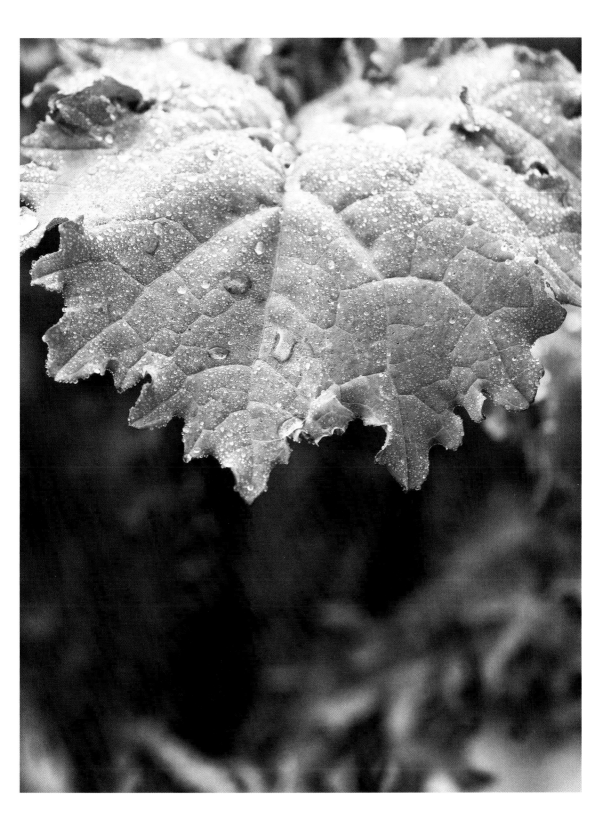

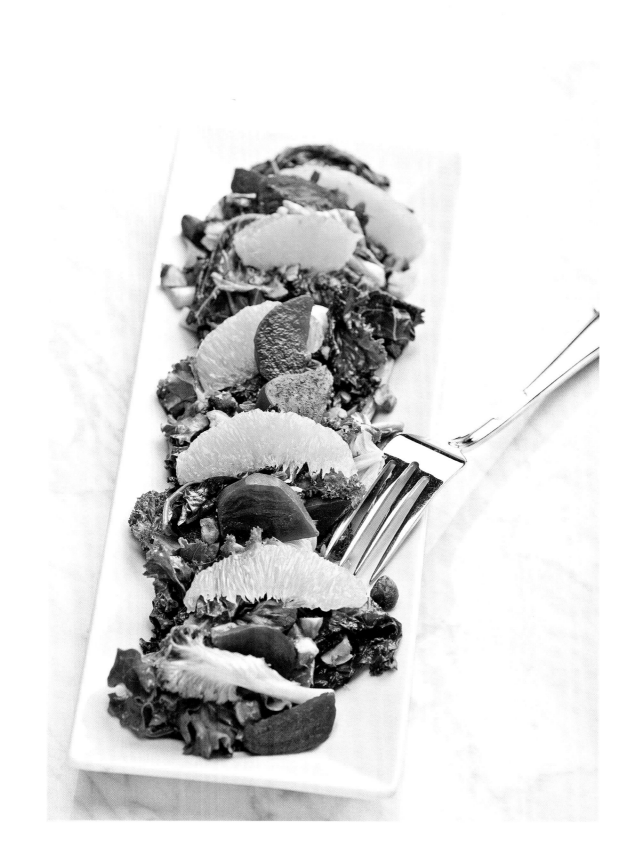

Warm Kale with Beets and Ginger

This warm salad, a decadent feast for the senses, is pure kale-rotica. Sexy, mood-boosting beets deliver a little happiness to your brain through a chemical called uridine, and the natural opioids in citrus protect you against pain (even the good kind). Top it all off with fresh ginger for a bit of spice . . . it doesn't get much more sensual. **Serves 4**

1 tablespoon extra virgin olive oil

1 tablespoon unsalted butter

2 tablespoons chopped fresh ginger

1 tablespoon brown sugar

2 medium oranges, zested and cut into segments

One 10-ounce bunch kale, trimmed and chopped (about 10 cups)

2 garlic cloves, chopped

4 beets, steamed and sliced (or one 15-ounce can sliced canned beets)

¼ cup chopped shelled pistachios or walnuts

➤ Heat a large skillet over medium heat. Add the olive oil, butter, ginger, garlic, brown sugar, and orange zest. Cook, stirring often, until the mixture becomes fragrant and the orange zest begins to brown, about 1 minute.

➤ Add the kale, press it down using a small metal lid, and cook for 2 to 3 minutes, stirring occasionally and continuing to press down with the lid until the kale wilts. Transfer to a large platter and top with the beets, orange segments, and pistachios. Serve immediately.

PER SERVING (2 CUPS): 223 calories, 6 g protein, 30 g carbohydrates, 10 g fat (2 g saturated), 7 mg cholesterol, 3 g fiber, 115 mg sodium

Black Bean Soup with Fresh Lime

This soup will heat you up and keep you warm all over. Limes possess a set of molecules that stimulate your opioid receptors, lighting up the pleasure center of your brain. Cayenne and chili powder contain capsaicin, a hunger-busting, immunity-building, euphoria-promoting compound that boosts your heart rate and increases blood flow . . . preparing you for the evening to come. **Serves 4**

2 tablespoons olive oil

1 small red onion, chopped
  (about 1 cup)

½ teaspoon salt

2 tablespoons ground cumin

2 tablespoons chili powder

¼ to ½ teaspoon ground cayenne

3 garlic cloves, minced

One 15-ounce can black beans,
  drained and rinsed

2 quarts low-sodium vegetable broth

One 10-ounce bunch kale, trimmed and
  thinly sliced (about 10 cups)

Zest of 1 lime

Juice of 2 limes

¼ cup chopped fresh cilantro

1 jalapeño or other chile, thinly sliced

➤ In a large saucepan, heat the olive oil over medium-high heat until hot but not smoking. Add the onion and salt. Cook, stirring often, until the onion becomes translucent and soft, 5 to 6 minutes. Add the cumin, chili powder, cayenne, and garlic. Continue to cook for 2 to 3 minutes, until the spices release their aroma. Increase the heat to high and add the beans and vegetable broth. Cover and bring to a boil.

➤ Reduce the heat to a simmer and continue cooking until the beans are tender and have started to break apart, about 20 minutes. Add the kale and cook for about 2 minutes more, stirring often, until the kale softens. Add the lime zest and juice. Top with the cilantro and jalapeño and serve immediately.

PER SERVING (2 CUPS): 172 calories, 11 g protein, 28 g carbohydrates, 4 g fat (5 g saturated), 5 mg cholesterol, 7 g fiber, 587 mg sodium

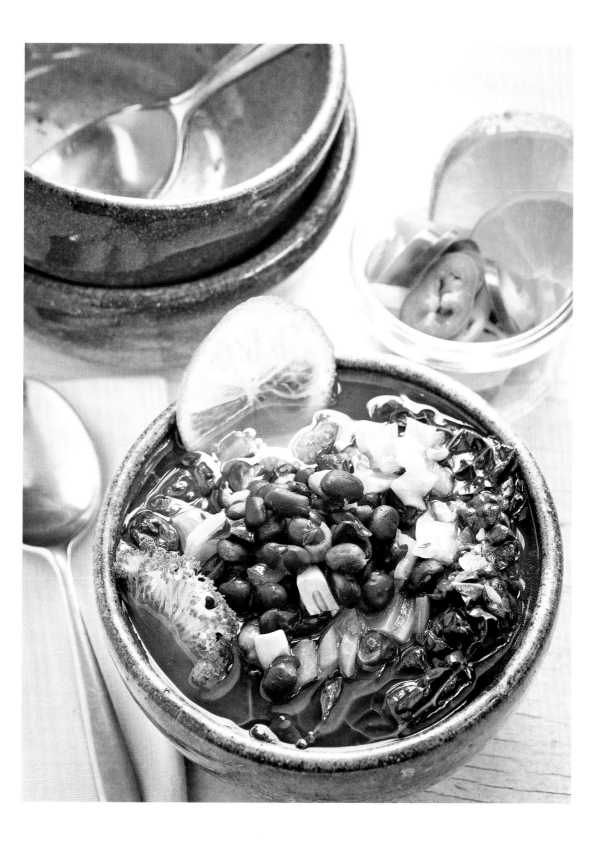

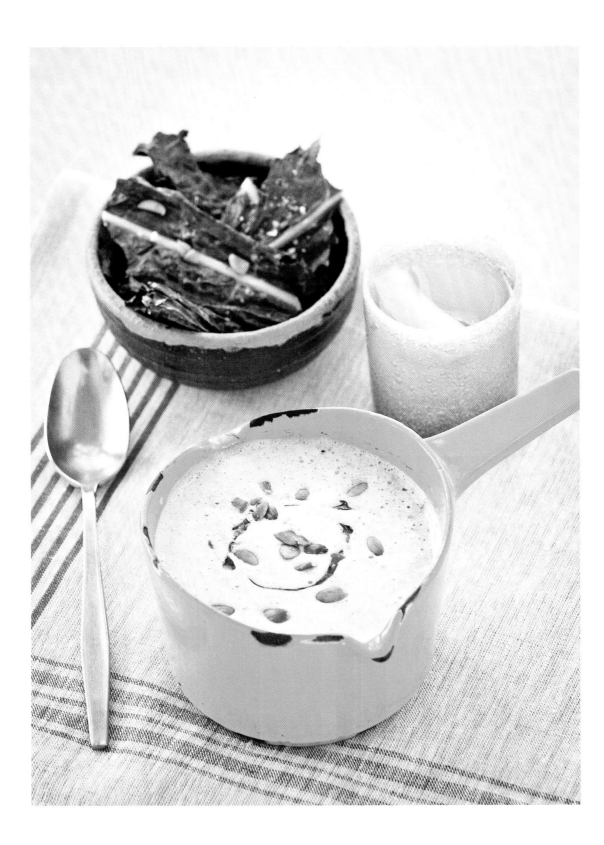

Cream of Kale Soup

Smooth, creamy foods are a sensual delight. You may feel a little naughty about using heavy cream in this healthy soup, but don't beat yourself up. The vitamin K and beta-carotene in kale are both fat-soluble compounds—so your body is more easily able to absorb them when you add a little healthy fat. Virtue never tasted so sinful. **Serves 4**

1 tablespoon olive oil

1 large red onion, sliced into thin rings

1 teaspoon brown sugar

½ teaspoon sea salt

One 10-ounce bunch kale, trimmed and roughly chopped (about 10 cups)

4 cups low-sodium vegetable broth

½ cup heavy cream

➤ Heat a large saucepan over medium heat. Add the olive oil, onion, sugar, and salt and cook for 10 to 15 minutes, stirring often, until the onion softens and starts to brown. Add the kale and vegetable broth, reduce the heat to low, and simmer for 1 to 2 minutes, until the kale begins to soften. Add the cream. Use an immersion blender, regular blender, or food processor to blend the soup until creamy. Divide among 4 bowls and serve immediately.

PER SERVING (3 CUPS): 232 calories, 5 g protein, 15 g carbohydrates, 18 g fat (8 g saturated), 47 mg cholesterol, 2 g fiber, 536 mg sodium

Sweet and Sour Veggies

In any steamy love affair, there are sweet and sour moments. Broccoli contains compounds known as glucosinolates, which are present in a variety of cruciferous vegetables and for some people can produce a bitter taste. Never fear—the orange marmalade and zest offer a hint of sweetness to balance this dish. Sweet, sour, and spice . . . these veggies are everything nice. **Serves 4**

---

1 cup short-grain brown rice

1 tablespoon canola oil

½ red bell pepper, cored, seeded, and cubed

1 cup broccoli florets

5 ounces kale, trimmed and chopped (about 5 cups)

¼ cup water

2 tablespoons reduced-sodium soy sauce

2 tablespoons low-sugar orange marmalade

4 teaspoons orange zest (from 1 large orange)

1 small jalapeño, seeded and thinly sliced

➤ Cook the rice according to the package instructions. Cover to keep warm and set aside.

➤ Place a large skillet over medium heat. Add the canola oil, along with the red pepper, broccoli, and kale. Reduce the heat to low and cook for 2 to 3 minutes, stirring often. Carefully add the water and cover. Steam for about 1 minute, until the veggies are fork tender. Turn the heat off and add the soy sauce and marmalade. Stir to coat. Transfer the rice into 4 bowls and top with orange zest and jalapeño. Top with the stir-fried vegetables and serve immediately.

PER SERVING (2 CUPS): 71 calories, 2 g protein, 8 g carbohydrates, 3 g fat (0 g saturated), 0 mg cholesterol, 1 g fiber, 304 mg sodium

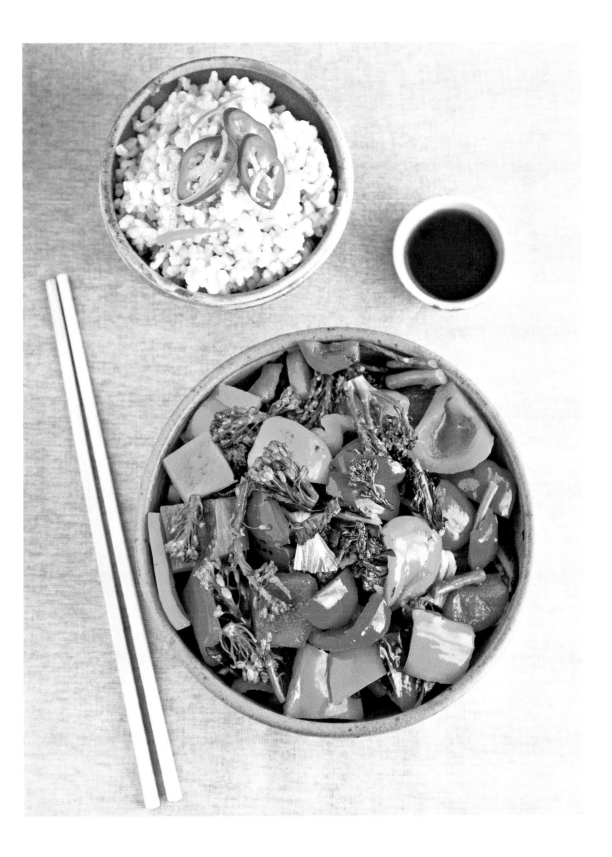

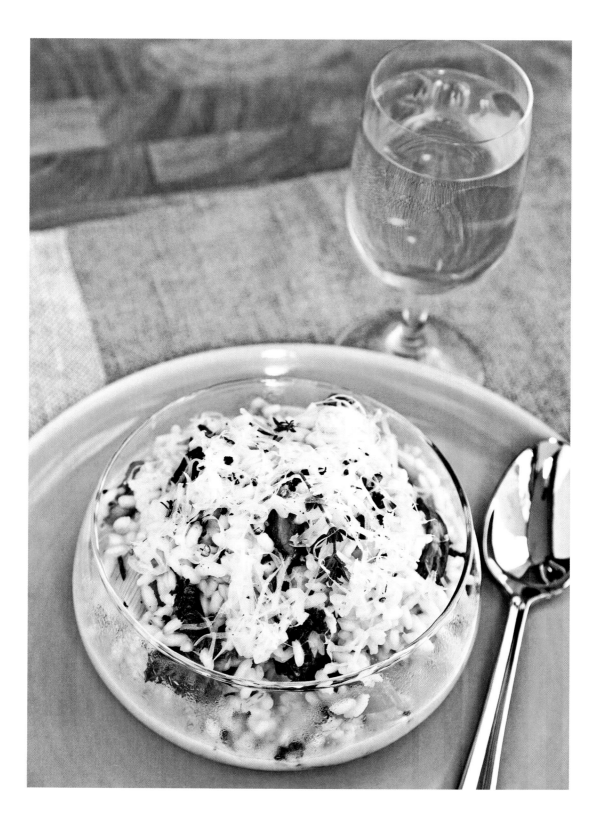

Mushroom and Kale Risotto

The mushrooms in this satisfying risotto lend the dish a deeply earthy, aromatic quality. Including mushrooms is a great way to add depth of flavor to many dishes for almost no calories. Mushrooms are high in selenium, a mineral that helps thyroid function and is also responsible for strong, shiny hair. **Serves 4**

4 cups low-sodium vegetable broth

1 tablespoon olive oil

½ pound assorted mushrooms, chopped

1 small onion or 2 leeks, white part only, chopped

4 garlic cloves, minced

1 tablespoon minced fresh thyme or rosemary

½ teaspoon sea salt

1 cup risotto rice, such as Arborio, Carnaroli, or Vialone Nano

1 cup dry white wine

5 ounces kale, trimmed and thinly sliced (about 5 cups)

½ cup grated or shaved Parmesan cheese

1 tablespoon unsalted butter

¼ teaspoon cracked black pepper

➤ Place the broth in a small saucepan over low heat. Heat a large skillet over medium heat and add the olive oil. Add the mushrooms, onion, garlic, thyme, and salt. Cook for 6 to 8 minutes, stirring often, until the mushrooms give off their liquid and the onion starts to soften. Add the rice and cook 1 minute more, stirring once or twice.

➤ Add the wine and cook for 1 to 2 minutes, stirring continuously, until the liquid is completely absorbed. Add ½ cup of the broth and cook at a hearty simmer until the broth is absorbed. Continue to add ½-cup amounts of the broth as the rice cooks, for a total of about 30 minutes, until the rice is softened but still al dente. Stir in half of the cheese and the butter. Sprinkle with the black pepper. Serve immediately with the remaining cheese.

PER SERVING (2 CUPS): 406 calories, 11 g protein, 54 g carbohydrates, 12 g fat (4 g saturated), 18 mg cholesterol, 3 g fiber, 500 mg sodium

Ramen Noodles with Kale

The mere mention of ramen noodles may bring you back to your college days . . . and just like then, it's time to experiment a little. This spicy ramen dish contains ginger, chiles, and garlic—aromatic spices that have two amazing properties: They help to increase blood flow throughout the body and help to protect your gut against harmful bacteria, as they work as natural antiseptics in your digestive tract.

Serves 4

1 tablespoon sesame oil

5 ounces shiitake mushrooms, stems removed, thinly sliced

4 garlic cloves, minced

One 1-inch piece ginger, peeled and minced

1 jalapeño chile, finely minced (seeds removed if you like it less spicy)

¼ teaspoon Chinese five-spice powder

One 10-ounce package Japanese curly noodles or chuka soba

1 cup low-sodium vegetable broth

4 cups chopped kale

1 tablespoon unsalted butter

2 scallions, chopped

➤ Heat a large skillet over medium-high heat. Add the sesame oil and mushrooms and cook for 1 to 2 minutes, stirring once or twice, until the mushrooms start to soften, adding 1 tablespoon of water if they begin to stick. Add the garlic, ginger, and chile and reduce the heat to medium. Cook for another 1 to 2 minutes, until the mushrooms are softened and the garlic is fragrant. Sprinkle in the five-spice powder and stir to coat. Add the noodles and vegetable broth.

➤ Cover, reduce the heat, and simmer for 4 to 5 minutes, until the noodles are tender. Add the kale and butter and cook for 1 to 2 minutes more, until the kale is wilted. Garnish with the scallions and serve immediately.

PER SERVING (2½ CUPS): 367 calories, 13 g protein, 68 g carbohydrates, 8 g fat (2 g saturated), 8 mg cholesterol, 3 g fiber, 625 mg sodium

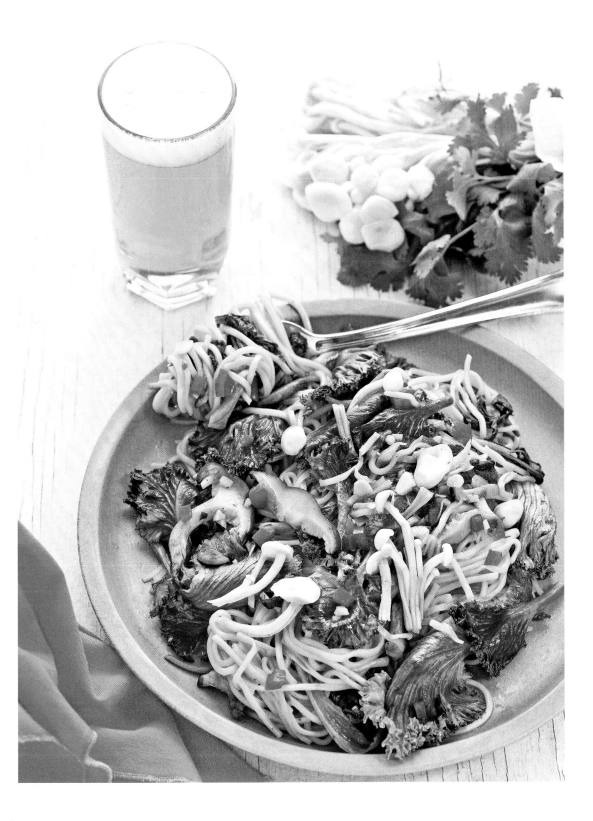

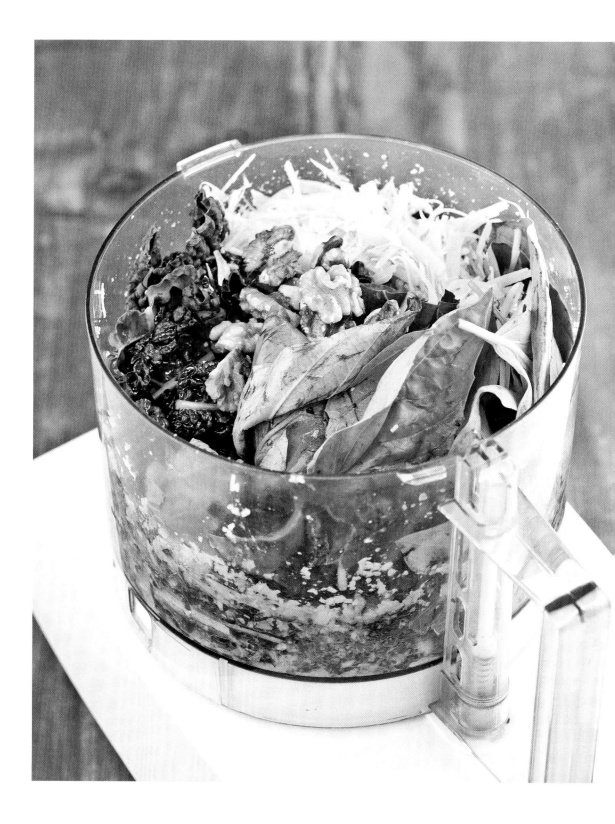

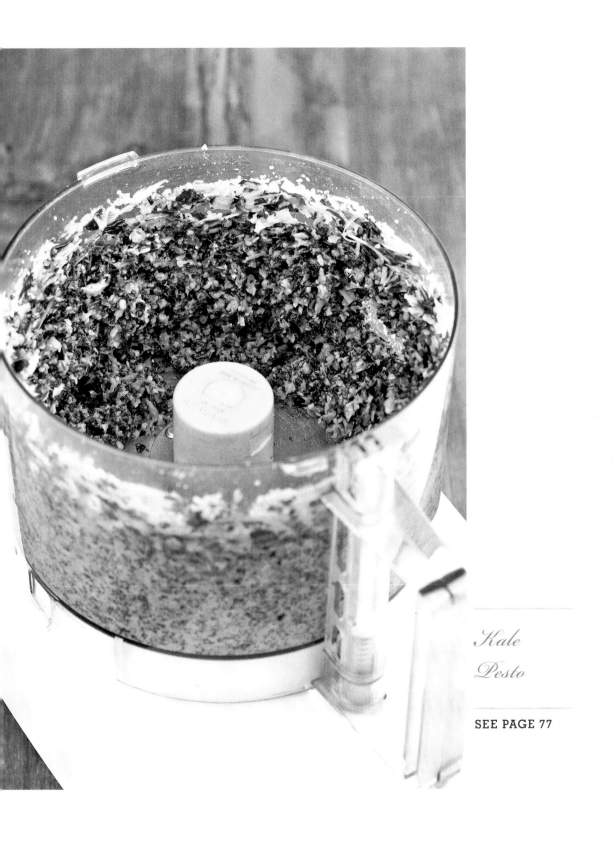

Kale
Pesto

SEE PAGE 77

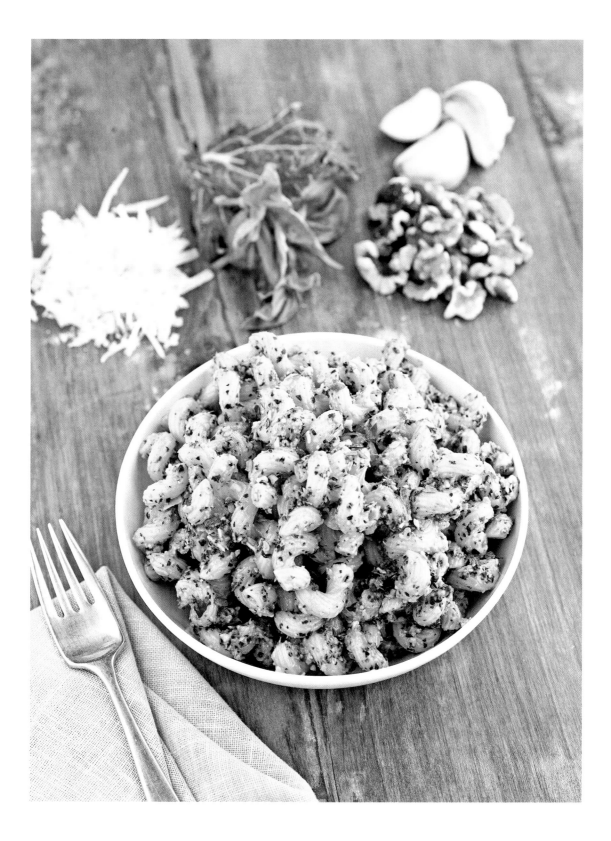

Kale Pesto with Toasted Walnuts

There is so much folate in this pesto, you'll make a pound of serotonin before bedtime, which means a night of great sleep and a smile in the morning. Both kale and walnuts feed your lover's brain with the omega-3 ALA, which is converted into molecules that protect your brain cells and are linked to a lower risk of depression. The pesto is equally delicious on pasta or brushed on grilled chicken. **Serves 8**

2 cups packed torn kale leaves, stems removed

1 cup packed fresh basil leaves

1 teaspoon sea salt

¼ cup extra virgin olive oil

¼ cup toasted walnuts

4 cloves garlic, chopped

½ cup grated Parmesan cheese

➤ In a food processor, combine the kale leaves, basil leaves, and salt. Pulse 10 to 12 times, until the kale leaves are finely chopped. With the motor running, drizzle in the olive oil. Scrape down the sides of the processor. Add the walnuts and garlic and process again, then add the cheese and pulse to combine. Toss with your favorite pasta and serve immediately.

PER SERVING (ABOUT ¼ CUP): 139 calories, 4 g protein, 3 g carbohydrates, 13 g fat (2 g saturated), 4 mg cholesterol, 1 g fiber, 279 mg sodium

Open Sesame

Rich, nutty, and exotic . . . the taste of sesame seeds, cultivated since the Bronze Age, will transport you to a distant land. Prized for its high oil and protein content, sesame is also high in the trace mineral copper, responsible for reducing inflammation in the joints. **Serves 4**

2 tablespoons sesame oil

1 teaspoon brown sugar

One 10-ounce bunch kale, trimmed and chopped (about 10 cups)

1 tablespoon unsalted butter

1 tablespoon toasted sesame seeds

➤ Heat a medium skillet over high heat. Add the sesame oil, brown sugar, and kale. Cook for about 2 minutes, pressing the kale down with a small saucepan lid until it wilts. Add the butter and stir until it melts. Sprinkle the sesame seeds over the top and serve immediately.

PER SERVING (1 CUP): 137 calories, 3 g protein, 8 g carbohydrates, 11 g fat (3 g saturated), 8 mg cholesterol, 2 g fiber, 31 mg sodium

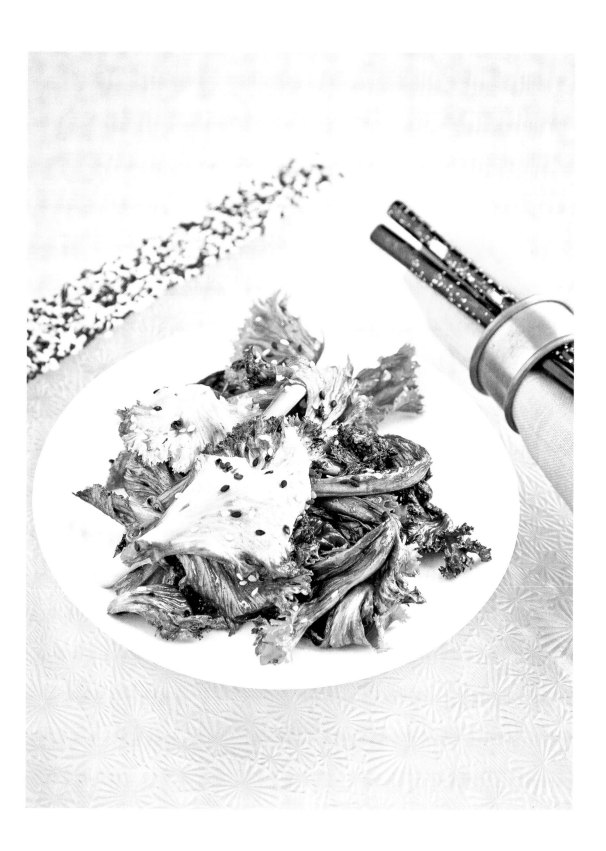

Green Pizza

Is there anything more tempting than a slice of hot pizza? Get your hands a little dirty by making your own pie at home. When tomatoes, basil, and cheese unite, it's not only a threesome made in taste heaven; these ingredients also offer the benefit of mood-boosting folate, important for protein metabolism and red blood cell production. **Serves 6**

1 pound whole wheat pizza dough, defrosted if frozen

One 28-ounce can diced tomatoes (such as San Marzano), drained

2 cups grated mozzarella cheese

¼ cup extra virgin olive oil, plus more for drizzling

1 cup packed torn kale leaves, including stems

¼ teaspoon salt

¼ cup packed fresh basil leaves

➤ Preheat the oven to 400°F.

➤ Roll the pizza dough into a 10-inch disk. Transfer to a 12-inch round pizza tin or shape into an 8 x 12-inch rectangle and transfer to a baking sheet.

➤ Scatter the diced tomatoes over the crust, leaving a 1-inch lip around the edge. Sprinkle with the mozzarella and drizzle with olive oil. Bake for 15 to 20 minutes, until the crust is golden and the cheese is bubbly.

➤ While the pizza is baking, prepare the kale drizzle. Combine the kale, olive oil, and salt in a food processor and pulse until a chunky green paste forms.

➤ Top the pie with the kale drizzle and the basil and cool for 5 minutes on the countertop. Cut into 12 wedges and serve immediately.

PER SERVING (2 SLICES): 370 calories, 20 g protein, 52 g carbohydrates, 10 g fat (4 g saturated), 20 mg cholesterol, 8 g fiber, 780 mg sodium

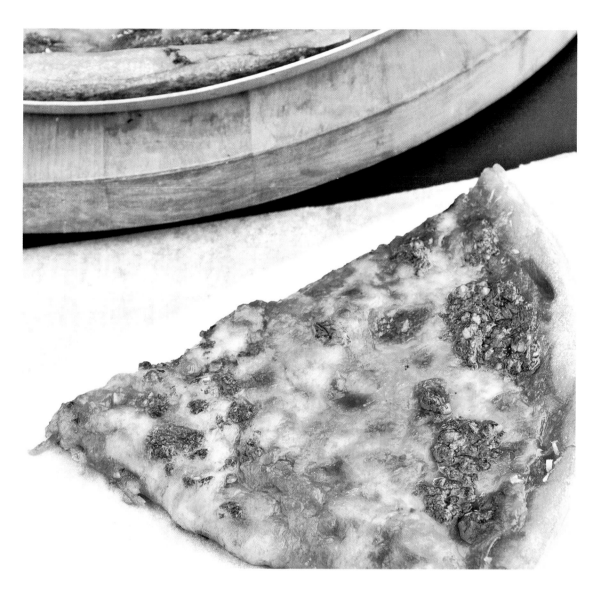

Did You Know? High-quality canned tomatoes not only make your dish taste better, they also offer nutritional benefits. Look for San Marzano tomatoes. Because they're grown in volcanic ash, they have more flavor and therefore may not contain as much added salt as other canned tomatoes.

Grains and Greens

Perfect partners are hard to find. But when they do come together, magic happens . . . like what occurs when you pair nutrient-dense quinoa with kale. It whispers, "Complete Protein, meet Miss Mega Vitamin." This double serving of iron will titillate your dopamine receptors—firing up your brain's pleasure centers.

Serves 4

1 cup quinoa, rinsed under cold water

1 tablespoon olive oil

One 10-ounce bunch kale, trimmed and chopped (about 10 cups)

3 cloves garlic, minced

½ teaspoon red chile flakes

2 cups low-sodium vegetable broth

One 4-ounce package goat cheese, at room temperature

Zest and juice of 1 lemon

½ teaspoon freshly grated nutmeg

¼ teaspoon salt

➤ Cook the quinoa according to the package instructions. Set aside.

➤ Heat a large skillet over high heat and add the olive oil. Add the kale, garlic, and red chile flakes and cook for 3 to 4 minutes, until the kale wilts. Add the broth and cook for another minute. Add the quinoa and cook for another minute, stirring once or twice until the quinoa is well mixed in. Cook for another minute, or until a third of the liquid is evaporated.

➤ Stir in the goat cheese, lemon zest, lemon juice, nutmeg, and salt. Serve immediately.

PER SERVING (2 CUPS): 429 calories, 15 g protein, 49 g carbohydrates, 16 g fat (6 g saturated), 18 mg cholesterol, 8 g fiber, 483 mg sodium

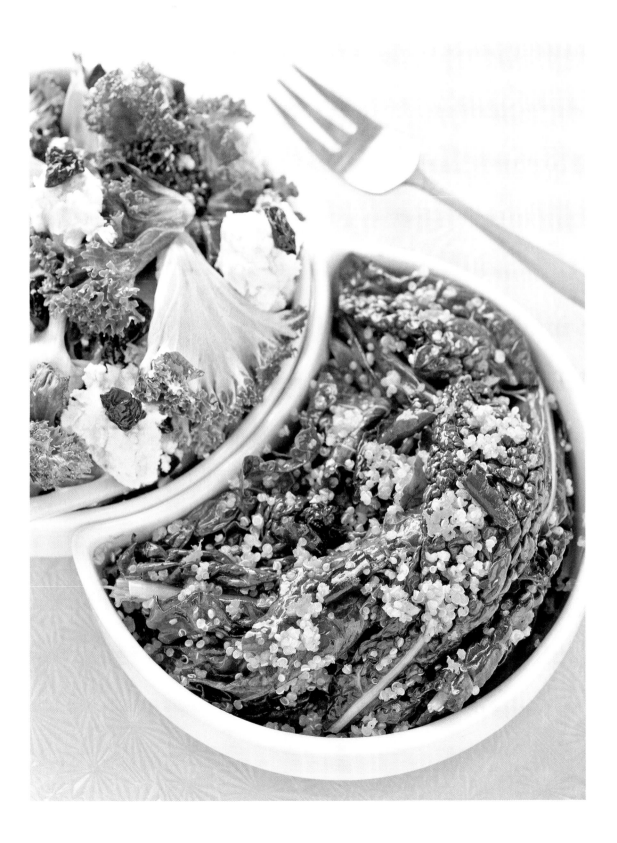

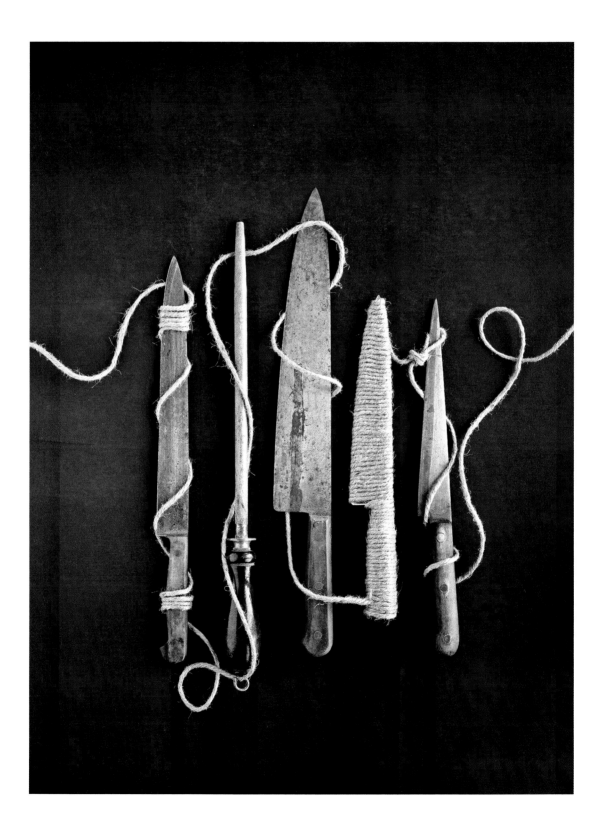

5.

Get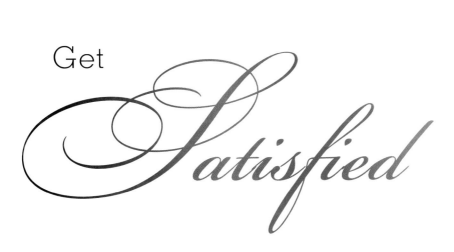

Thai'd Up Shrimp

When it comes to seafood . . . go wild. Choosing wild shrimp is a great way to incorporate seafood into your diet—it's lower in mercury and other toxins than large fish like tuna and offers several essential nutrients, including astaxanthin, a powerful anti-inflammatory compound that helps to promote brain health. **Serves 4**

---

8 ounces wide rice noodles

⅓ cup lime juice

⅓ cup water

4 teaspoons fish sauce

1 tablespoon rice vinegar

1 tablespoon granulated sugar

2 teaspoons chili sauce, such as Sriracha

2 tablespoons olive oil

2 garlic cloves, finely minced

1 shallot, finely minced

½ pound peeled and deveined wild shrimp

2 eggs, lightly beaten

¼ cup toasted walnuts, roughly chopped

2 cups bean sprouts

4 scallions, thinly sliced

5 ounces kale, trimmed and chopped (about 5 cups)

½ cup packed chopped cilantro leaves

➤ Place the noodles in a heatproof bowl and add boiling water to cover. Soak for 20 minutes, or until softened but not mushy. Drain and set aside.

➤ In a small bowl, whisk together the lime juice, water, fish sauce, rice vinegar, sugar, chili sauce, and 1 tablespoon oil. Set aside.

➤ Heat 1 tablespoon oil in a large skillet over medium-high heat. Add the garlic, shallot, and shrimp and cook for 3 to 4 minutes, until the shrimp is pink and cooked through. Add the eggs, stir, and scramble until just moist.

➤ Add the cooked noodles, lime juice mixture, walnuts, sprouts, and scallions. Using a pair of tongs or 2 large spoons, toss until the noodles are evenly coated. Add the kale and cook, tossing constantly, until the noodles are tender and the sauce has thickened slightly, 3 to 4 minutes more. Add the cilantro and serve immediately.

PER SERVING (2½ CUPS): 392 calories, 10 g protein, 62 g carbohydrates, 12 g fat (2 g saturated), 93 mg cholesterol, 3 g fiber, 688 mg sodium

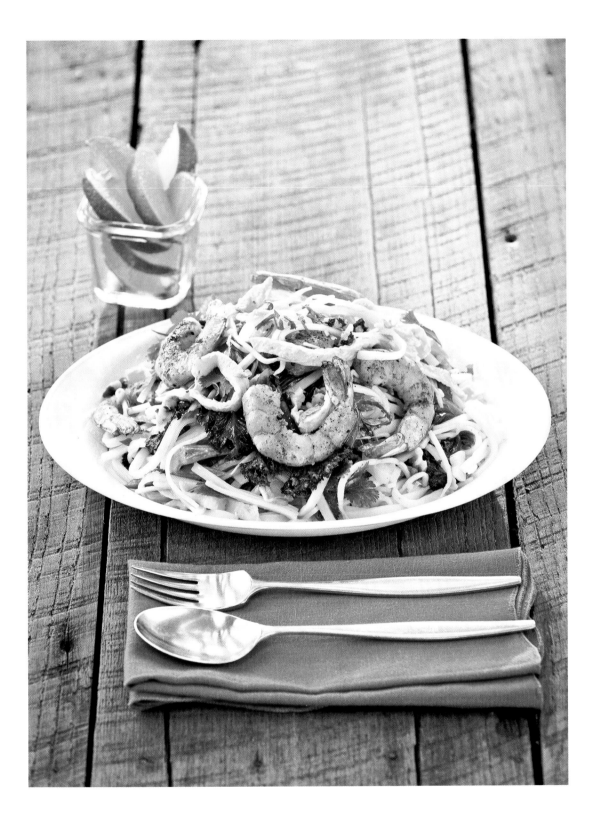

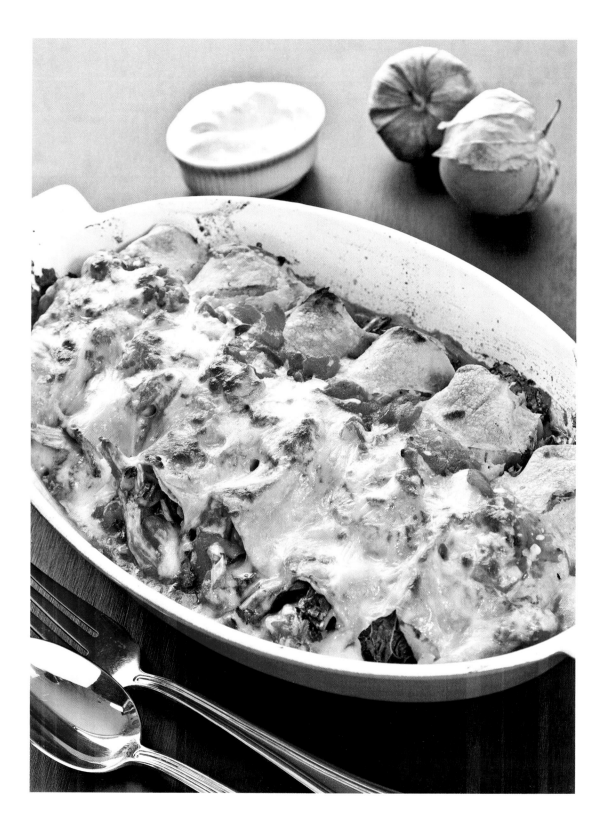

Chicken Enchiladas

You've always wanted the whole enchilada, and now you can have it. No need to be ashamed of a big appetite—adding kale to your dish ensures that the portion size is large enough to satisfy without packing on calories, and gives you some fiber to boot. Sprinkle on even more jalapeños for extra heat—and an extra dose of vitamin C. **Serves 4**

1 tablespoon olive oil

1 small yellow or white onion, chopped

1 large jalapeño, seeded and chopped

1 large garlic clove, chopped

One 15-ounce can chopped tomatoes

5 ounces kale, trimmed and chopped (about 5 cups)

2 skinless, boneless, free-range organic chicken breasts (about 12 ounces), cooked and thinly sliced

½ teaspoon dried oregano

8 small (6-inch) soft corn tortillas

¼ cup sour cream (organic if possible)

2 cups grated mozzarella cheese (organic if possible)

½ cup jarred salsa verde, optional

➤ Preheat the oven to 400°F.

➤ Heat a large skillet over medium-high heat. Add the olive oil, then add the onion, jalapeño, and garlic. Cook for 5 to 7 minutes, stirring occasionally, until the onion begins to soften but not brown. Remove from the heat and add the tomatoes along with their juices, the kale, chicken, and oregano. Stir until the tomato juices coat the chicken and kale.

➤ Set out an 8 x 12-inch baking dish. Wrap ½ cup of the chicken mixture in each tortilla and lay the tortillas seam side down in the baking dish. Spoon the sour cream over the tops of the tortillas and sprinkle with the cheese. Bake uncovered for 10 to 15 minutes, until the cheese begins to brown and the filling is warm. Serve immediately with salsa verde if desired.

PER SERVING (2 ENCHILADAS): 420 calories, 36 g protein, 26 g carbohydrates, 21 g fat (9 g saturated), 92 mg cholesterol, 3 g fiber, 518 mg sodium

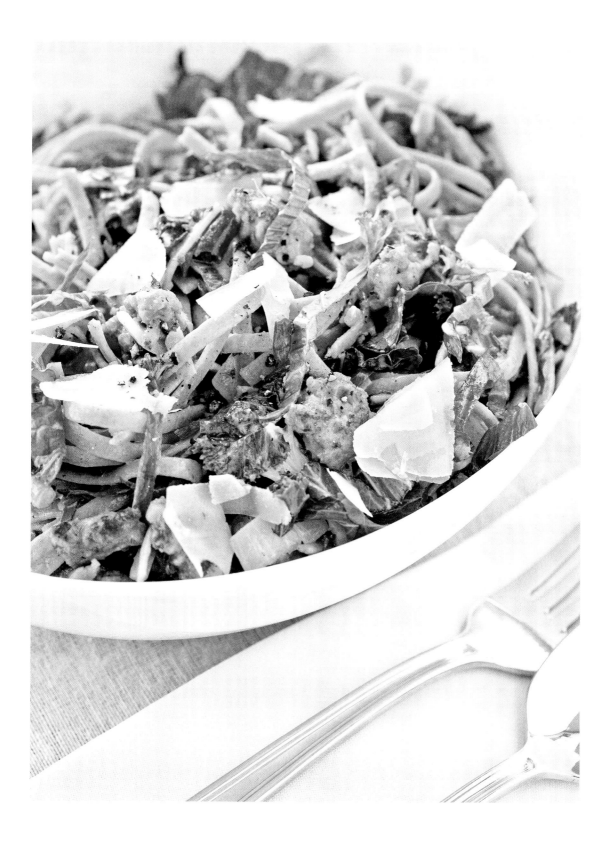

Linguine with Sausage and Kale

If you haven't been satisfied in a long time, this dish is sure to please. Flavorful sausage is high in thiamine, a vitamin needed for long bursts of vitality. And whole wheat pasta keeps your blood sugar stable while supplying you with plenty of energy. Just call it the dinner of champions. **Serves 4**

2 tablespoons kosher salt

½ pound whole wheat linguine (preferably fresh)

1 tablespoon olive oil

3 links sweet Italian sausage

1 teaspoon red pepper flakes

½ yellow or red onion, chopped

One 10-ounce bunch kale, trimmed and chopped (about 10 cups)

¼ cup heavy cream

½ cup freshly grated or shaved Parmesan cheese

➤ Bring a large saucepan of water to a boil. Add the salt and pasta and cook according to the package instructions. Drain the pasta, reserving 1 cup of the cooking water.

➤ Heat a large skillet over medium heat and add the oil. Add the sausage and cook for 2 to 3 minutes, breaking it up with the back of a spoon. Sprinkle ½ teaspoon of the red pepper flakes over the sausage and press them into the meat. Add the onion and cook for 2 minutes more, or until the onion softens. Add the kale and reduce the heat to low. Cook for 2 minutes more, stirring often, until the kale is tender.

➤ Add the cream and scrape up any bits of sausage clinging to the inside bottom of the pan. Add the linguine and half of the cheese and toss well. Add half of the reserved pasta water and toss again, adding more if the mixture is too dry. Divide the pasta among 4 plates or bowls and garnish with remaining ½ teaspoon red pepper flakes and the cheese.

PER SERVING (ABOUT 2½ CUPS): 430 calories, 18 g protein, 53 g carbohydrates, 18 g fat (7 g saturated), 35 mg cholesterol, 6 g fiber, 510 mg sodium

Steak Fajitas

Want a hard body? Protein is essential for the formation of new muscle tissue, and these steak fajitas do double duty, since kale is one of the few high-protein vegetables. Both steak and kale are also good sources of iron, and when paired together help to increase iron absorption in your body. In this case, one plus one equals three. It's a ménage à trois of healthy benefits. **Serves 4**

1 pound grass-fed flank steak

2 teaspoons mild or hot chili powder

1 teaspoon ground cumin

½ teaspoon sea salt

2 tablespoons canola oil

1 large yellow onion, sliced

2 red or orange bell peppers, cored, seeded, and sliced lengthwise into strips

5 ounces kale leaves, trimmed (about 5 cups)

½ cup chopped fresh cilantro, including stems

8 small (8-inch) whole wheat soft tortillas

1 cup grated cheese, such as pepper Jack or Colby (organic if possible), optional

1 lime, quartered

➤ Season the steak with the chili powder, cumin, and salt. Heat a large skillet over medium-high heat. Add 1 tablespoon of the canola oil and the steak. Cook for 18 to 20 minutes, turning once or twice, until the steak is browned and medium-rare inside. Set aside.

➤ In the same skillet, add the remaining 1 tablespoon canola oil along with the onion and bell peppers. Cook for 2 to 3 minutes, stirring often, until the peppers soften. Add the kale and cook for 1 minute more, until the leaves start to soften. Turn off the heat and cover.

➤ Thinly slice the flank steak against the grain into 16 slices. Place 2 pieces of the steak into each tortilla. Divide the pepper and kale mixture among the tortillas and top each with cilantro and 2 tablespoons of cheese, if using. Serve immediately with lime wedges.

PER SERVING (2 FILLED SOFT TORTILLAS): 397 calories, 25 g protein, 45 g carbohydrates, 13 g fat (3 g saturated), 251 mg cholesterol, 7 g fiber, 489 mg sodium

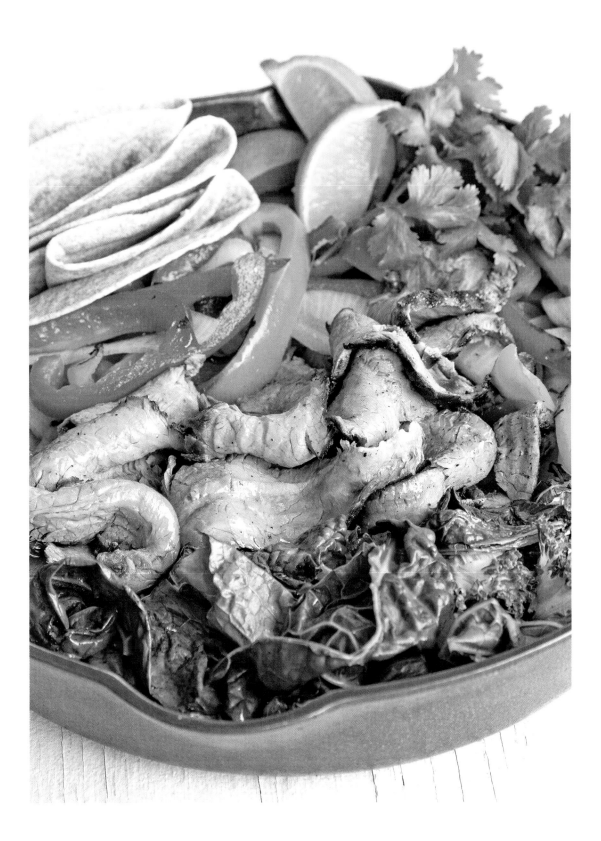

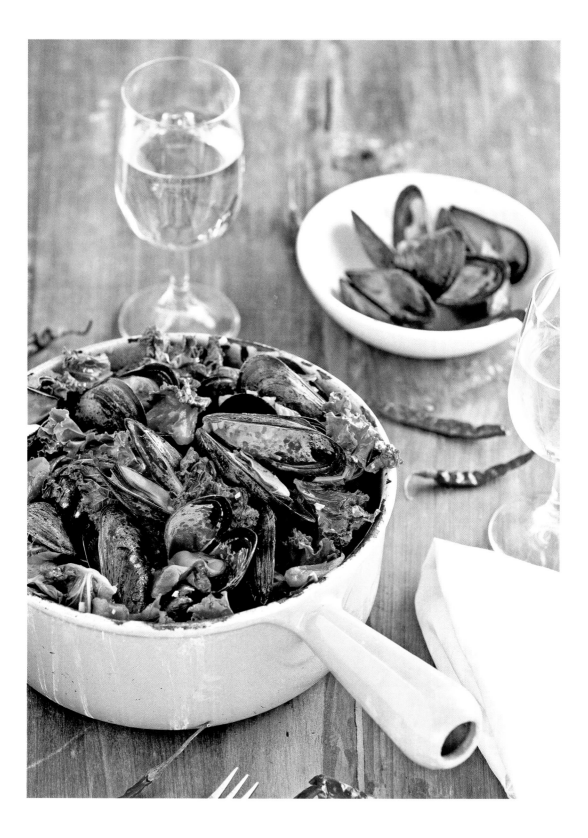

Spicy Mussels with Kale

When you combine mussels with fresh chiles, you'd better be prepared for a raucous night ahead—both ingredients are known aphrodisiacs. Apart from sheer sex appeal, there's another reason to dig in: Mussels provide one of the most highly concentrated sources of vitamin B$_{12}$, which plays a significant role in regulating metabolism and energy production. And at just 100 calories for every fifteen mussels, you can dig in without sin. **Serves 4**

2 pounds tightly closed raw mussels

1 tablespoon olive oil

4 garlic cloves, thinly sliced

1 small chile, such as habanero or serrano, minced, seeds removed

One 10-ounce bunch kale, trimmed and thinly sliced (about 10 cups)

½ cup white wine

One 15-ounce can diced tomatoes, drained

¼ teaspoon salt

⅛ teaspoon freshly ground black pepper

¼ cup chopped fresh flat-leaf parsley

➤ Place the mussels in a large bowl of cold water and soak them for 15 to 20 minutes. With your fingers or a slotted spoon, lift the mussels out of the water and place them in a colander. Rinse under cold running water several times and discard any mussels that are open. Check each mussel for a threadlike string hanging out of the shell (called the beard). To remove the beard, use a tea towel to take hold of the beard, pull firmly toward the hinge end of the shell, and tug it free.

➤ Heat a large saucepan or sauté pan with sides over medium-high heat. Add the olive oil, garlic, and chile. Reduce the heat to medium-low and cook for 1 minute, stirring occasionally, until the garlic becomes fragrant.

➤ Add the mussels, kale, wine, diced tomatoes, salt, and pepper. Cover and cook for 3 to 4 minutes more, shaking the pan, until the mussels open and the meat inside is cooked through. Discard any mussels that have not opened. Sprinkle with the parsley and serve immediately.

PER SERVING (¾ POUND MUSSELS PLUS SAUCE WITH KALE): 329 calories, 30 g protein, 22 g carbohydrates, 8 g fat (1 g saturated), 63 mg cholesterol, 2 g fiber, 858 mg sodium

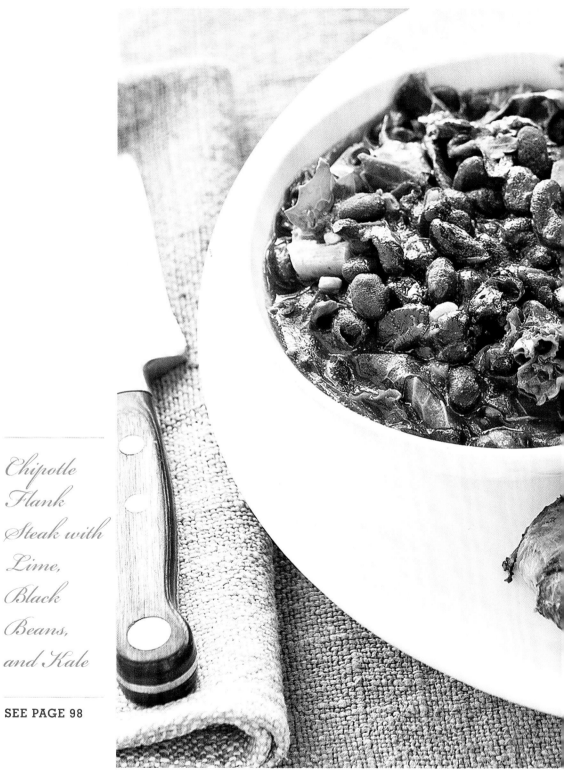

Chipotle Flank Steak with Lime, Black Beans, and Kale

SEE PAGE 98

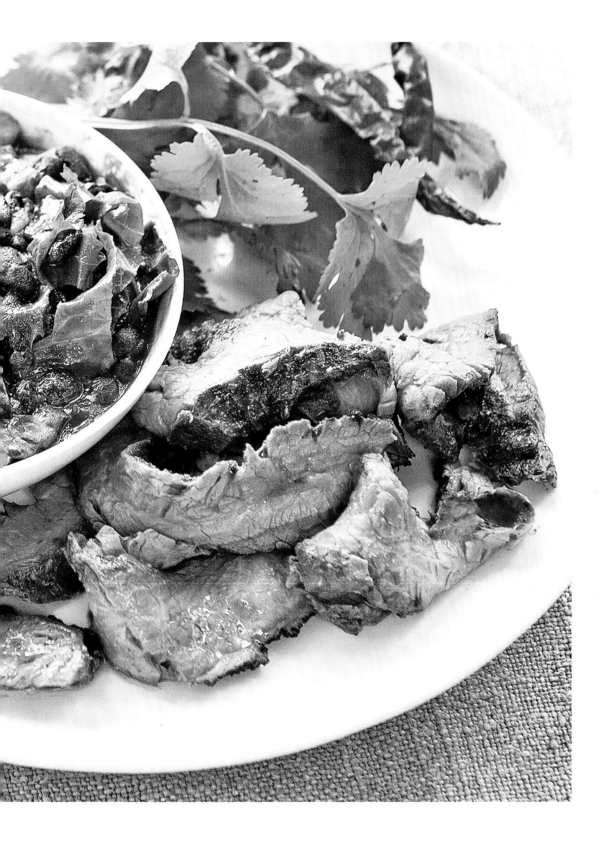

Chipotle Flank Steak with Lime, Black Beans, and Kale

This sizzling south-of-the-border dish will turn an ordinary weeknight into a red-hot fiesta. The combination of flavorful flank steak and black beans contains more than half of your daily iron needs, giving your muscles the fuel they need for a serious workout. The smokiness and heat of the chipotle chiles will tingle your lips and add some swagger to your hips. **Serves 4**

1 pound grass-fed flank steak

1 tablespoon chopped chipotle chiles in adobo sauce

¼ teaspoon sea salt

1 tablespoon olive oil

4 garlic cloves, minced

Olive oil cooking spray

1 cup Simple Chicken Broth (page 108)

One 15-ounce can black beans, drained and well rinsed

1 teaspoon mild chili powder

One 10-ounce bunch kale, trimmed and chopped (about 10 cups)

½ cup packed chopped fresh cilantro

Zest and juice of 1 lime

➤ Rub the steak with the chipotle chiles and sprinkle both sides with the salt. Place the steak inside a zipper-lock bag along with the olive oil and garlic.

Seal and refrigerate for at least 1 hour or overnight.

➤ Heat a grill or grill pan over medium-high heat. Coat with cooking spray and place the steak on the grill. Cook for 8 to 10 minutes per side, turning occasionally, for a total of 20 minutes, until the steak is medium-rare, or 25 minutes for medium. Rest steak on a cutting board for at least 5 minutes to allow the juices to redistribute.

➤ Meanwhile, combine the chicken broth, black beans, and chili powder in a large saucepan. Place over low heat, bring to a simmer, and simmer for 4 to 5 minutes, until the beans are warm. Add the kale, cover, and cook for 2 to 3 minutes, stirring often, until the kale wilts. Add the cilantro and lime zest and juice and serve immediately with the sliced flank steak.

PER SERVING (4 OUNCES FLANK STEAK, 1 CUP BLACK BEANS): 320 calories, 31 g protein, 24 g carbohydrates, 13 g fat (4 g saturated), 53 mg cholesterol, 7 g fiber, 603 mg sodium

Did You Know? Sea salt is like a kiss from the ocean, with a superior taste and texture to the commercially produced variety that make it perfect for cooking. In addition to containing essential trace minerals, some sea salts are lower in sodium than traditional table salt.

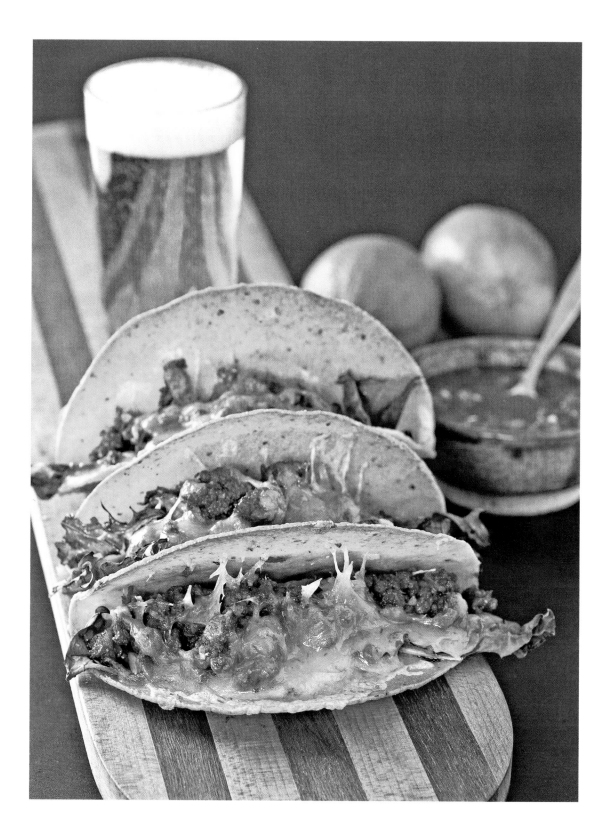

Beef and Kale Tacos

Are you in love with a hard-core carnivore who simply won't touch the green stuff? Well, here's the perfect way to get your sweetie to eat less meaty. He'll never notice the veggies in this beef lover's delight. He probably also won't notice that the meat in his taco contains zinc, niacin, and vitamin B$_{12}$, essential vitamins and minerals for robust health. Shh . . . it'll be our little secret. **Serves 4**

1 tablespoon olive oil

½ pound ground grass-fed beef

2 carrots, grated

2 garlic cloves, chopped

½ teaspoon sea salt

1 tablespoon mild chili powder

1 teaspoon ground cumin

2 tablespoons tomato paste

1 cup water

12 corn taco shells

2 cups kale leaves sliced into thin strips

1 cup shredded cheddar or pepper Jack cheese (organic if possible)

12 teaspoons jarred salsa

➤ Preheat the oven to 300°F.

➤ Heat a large skillet over medium-high heat. Add the olive oil, then add the beef, carrots, and garlic. Sprinkle with the salt. Cook for 4 to 5 minutes, stirring occasionally, until meat begins to brown and the vegetables soften. Add the chili powder, cumin, and tomato paste. Cook for an additional 1 to 2 minutes, until the spices become fragrant. Add the water, reduce the heat, and simmer for 4 to 5 minutes, until the beef is no longer pink in the center.

➤ Meanwhile, place the taco shells in the oven for 5 to 10 minutes to warm them (or warm them in the toaster oven). Assemble each taco by spooning in 2 tablespoons of the meat and some of the kale and cheese into each shell. Top each taco with 1 teaspoon salsa and serve immediately.

PER SERVING (3 TACOS): 386 calories, 24 g protein, 30 g carbohydrates, 17 g fat (5 g saturated), 45 mg cholesterol, 3 g fiber, 710 mg sodium

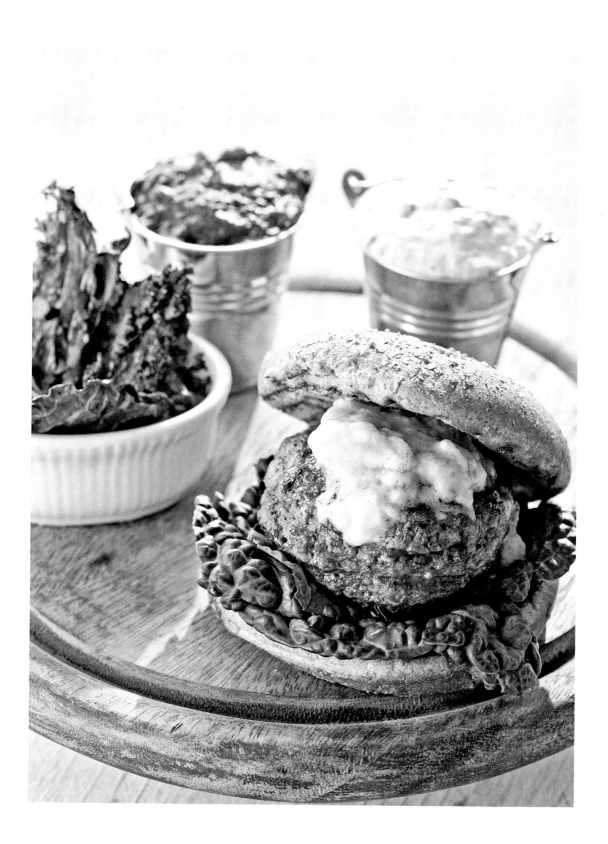

Beef Burger with Grilled Kale

You've been doing it in the car when nobody's looking . . . but you don't have to hide anymore. It's time to come clean—and this finger-licking-good burger is so much more satisfying than those greasy drive-through hockey pucks. Plus grass-fed beef is leaner and lower in calories than conventional beef. It even contains a unique fat that may help prevent cancer, diabetes, and heart disease. Talk about an afternoon delight. **Serves 4**

1 pound grass–fed ground sirloin

4 teaspoons barbecue or steak sauce

¼ teaspoon sea salt

½ cup crumbled blue cheese

4 large kale leaves

4 whole grain or whole wheat burger
  buns, split

➤ Place the sirloin, barbecue sauce, and salt in a large bowl. Using your fingers, mix well and form the mixture into 4 patties.

➤ Fire up the grill or heat a large grill pan over high heat. Grill the burgers for 10 to 15 minutes, until they are browned on the outside but still slightly pink (but not translucent) on the inside. Top each burger with 2 tablespoons of the blue cheese. Transfer the burgers to a plate and tent with aluminum foil to keep warm. Add the kale to the grill and grill for 2 to 3 minutes, turning often, until it is soft. Remove kale leaves from grill. Grill the bun halves for 30 seconds, cut side down. Remove from grill. Assemble burgers, placing grilled kale on bottom bun with the burger and top bun on top. Serve immediately.

PER SERVING (1 BURGER TOPPED WITH KALE PLUS BUN): 347 calories, 34 g protein, 28 g carbohydrates, 12 g fat (6 g saturated), 82 mg cholesterol, 4 g fiber, 642 mg sodium

Did You Know? If you can't find grass-fed ground sirloin, you can substitute lean grass-fed beef cubes and grind them yourself at home using a food processor or the grinder attachment on your mixer.

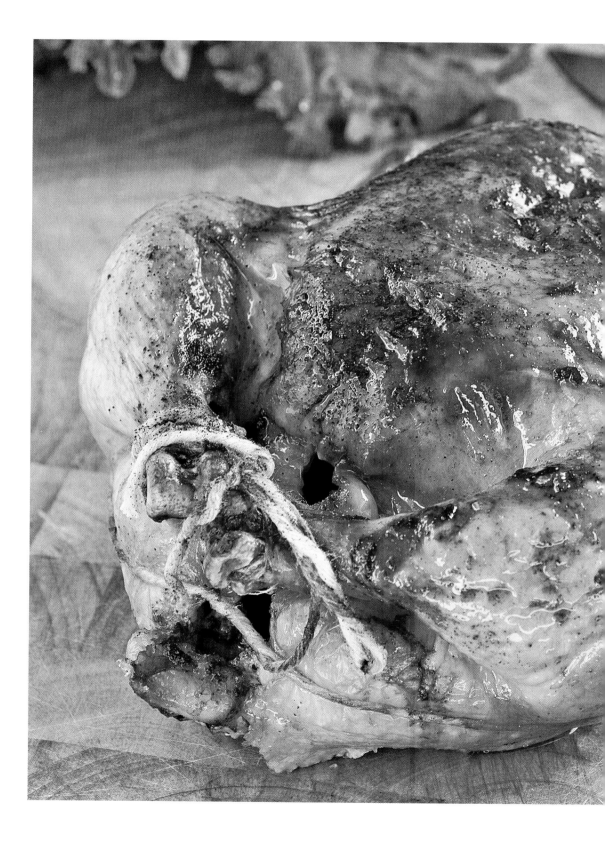

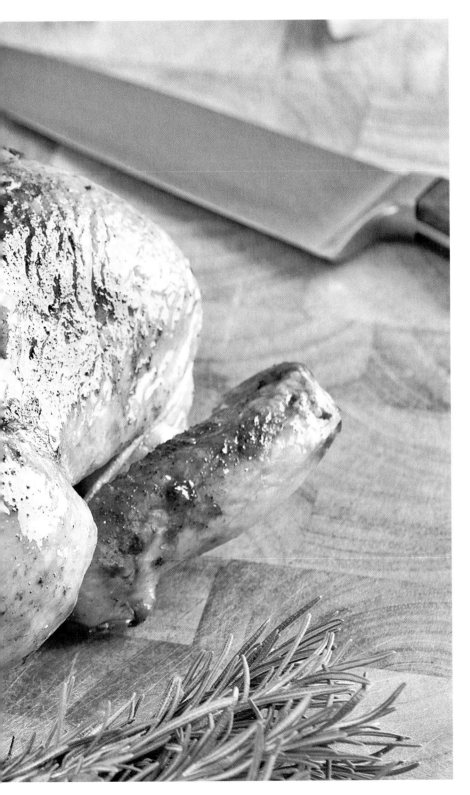

Roasted
Chicken
and
Kale

SEE PAGE 106

Roasted Chicken and Kale

There's nothing like a perfectly roasted chicken. This recipe couldn't be any easier—just lay your chicken down on the countertop, tie her legs firmly together, and rub her down with butter and lemon. Allow her to cook slowly in the oven and your patience will be rewarded with the most juicy, succulent meat. Lift her onto a bed of kale for a complete and satisfying meal. Chicken is a great source of lean protein, keeping your muscles toned and providing satisfaction that lasts. **Serves 4**

One 3½-pound free-range organic
   roasting chicken

1½ teaspoons sea salt

3 lemons, cut into wedges

1 sprig fresh rosemary

1 tablespoon unsalted butter, softened

¼ teaspoon freshly ground black pepper

1 tablespoon fresh thyme leaves

½ cup water

One 10-ounce bunch kale, trimmed
   and thinly sliced (about 10 cups)

1 tablespoon olive oil

➤ Preheat the oven to 400°F.

➤ Line a shallow roasting pan with aluminum foil and place a roasting rack or small wire cookie rack inside. Rinse the chicken well under cold running water and pat dry with paper towels. Season the inside of the cavity with 1 teaspoon of the salt and fill with half of the lemon wedges and the rosemary sprig.

➤ Truss or tie the chicken legs with a piece of cotton kitchen twine. Rub the chicken with the butter and squeeze the remaining lemon wedges over the surface of the chicken. Sprinkle with black pepper and thyme leaves. Add water to the bottom of the roasting pan. Roast the chicken uncovered for 1½ to 2 hours, until the meat reaches an internal temperature of 170°F and the meat surrounding the thigh joint is no longer pink. Remove the chicken from the oven and allow it to rest for 5 minutes to give the juices time to redistribute before carving.

➤ While the chicken is resting, prepare the kale. Place the kale in a large bowl along with the olive oil and toss well. Spread the kale out on an ungreased baking sheet. Sprinkle with remaining ½ teaspoon of salt. Transfer to the oven and bake for 10 minutes, or until the kale begins to brown around the edges and is cooked through.

➤ Carve the chicken and remove the skin. Scrape off the lemon and rosemary clinging to the skin and transfer to a platter. Discard the skin and slice the meat. Serve with the roasted kale.

PER SERVING (¼ POUND CHICKEN PLUS 2 CUPS KALE): 284 calories, 40 g protein, 17 g carbohydrates, 9 g fat (3 g saturated), 127 mg cholesterol, 5 g fiber, 360 mg sodium

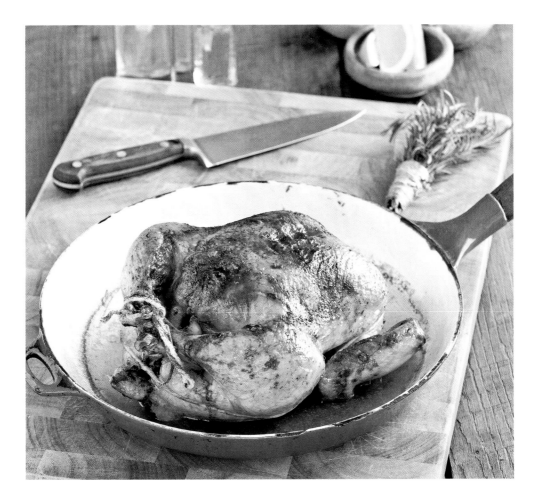

Simple Chicken Broth

Tired of faking it? Then break up with canned chicken broth for good—it will never deliver what you need. Most packaged broth contains preservatives, artificial colorings, and a ton of sodium—which can leave you bloated, dehydrated, and decidedly unsexy. Spend a little time simmering the real thing at home and you'll be rewarded with a rich depth of flavor and a much healthier stock. You can strain the vegetables, if you prefer. **Makes 2 quarts**

1 free-range organic chicken breast on the bone, with skin (about 6 ounces)

½ teaspoon sea salt

1 teaspoon olive oil

1 large red onion, chopped

2 medium carrots, chopped

2 stalks celery, chopped

8 kale stems (leftover from the Roasted Kale Chips recipe on page 42)

¼ cup chopped fresh parsley

1 teaspoon whole black peppercorns

2 bay leaves

2 quarts water

➤ Sprinkle the chicken with the salt. Heat a large saucepan over medium heat. Add the chicken skin side down and cook for 3 to 4 minutes, turning once or twice, until it is well browned. Add the onion, carrots, celery, and kale stems and cook for 3 to 4 minutes more, stirring occasionally, until the vegetables soften.

➤ Add the parsley, peppercorns, bay leaves, and water. Bring to a gentle boil over high heat, then immediately reduce the heat to low, cover, and simmer for 20 to 25 minutes, skimming the top of the broth with a spoon as any foam or fat gathers. Remove the chicken and discard the skin. Reserve the meat for chicken noodle soup.

➤ Cool completely, then store in an airtight container and refrigerate for up to 1 week, or store in the freezer for up to 6 months.

PER SERVING (1 CUP INCLUDING VEGETABLES): 40 calories, 0 g protein, 4 g carbohydrates, 2 g fat (0 g saturated), 1 mg cholesterol, 1 g fiber, 125 mg sodium

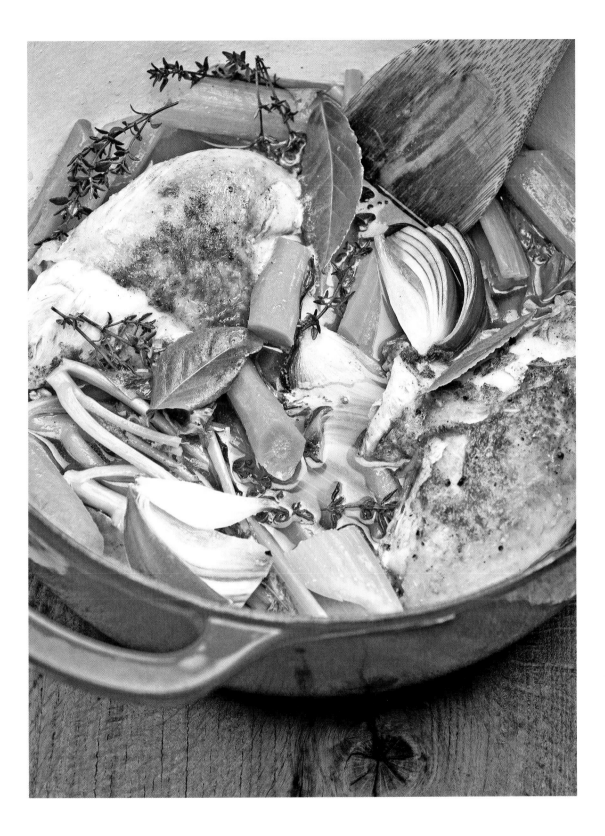

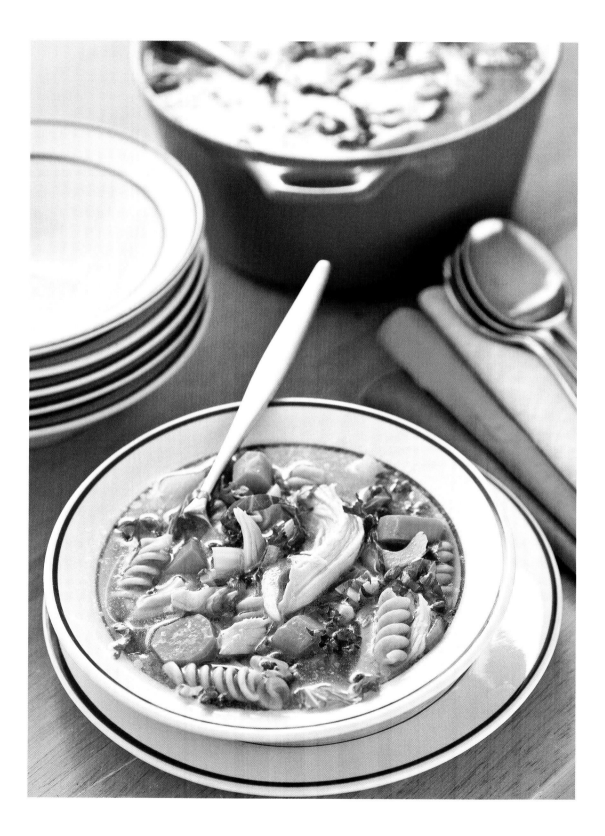

Kale Chicken Noodle Soup

Sometimes there's nothing more enticing than a wholesome, all-American classic. This chicken noodle soup made with simple ingredients will nourish you, body *and* soul. And thanks to the addition of kale, each serving offers a tremendous amount of beta-carotene and vitamin C, which will help keep you healthy and vibrant all winter long. **Serves 8**

---

8 ounces whole wheat pasta, such as penne or shells

1 free-range organic chicken breast on the bone, with skin (about 6 ounces)

1½ teaspoons sea salt

¼ teaspoon freshly ground black pepper

1 tablespoon olive oil

2 medium carrots, thinly sliced

2 stalks celery, thinly sliced

1 large red onion, chopped

4 quarts water

One 10-ounce bunch kale, trimmed and chopped (about 10 cups)

➤ Cook the pasta according to the package instructions. Drain and set aside.

➤ Sprinkle the chicken with the salt and pepper. Heat a large stockpot over medium-high heat. Add the olive oil, then the chicken skin side down, followed by the carrots, celery, and onion. Cook for 4 to 5 minutes, stirring often, until the vegetables soften and the chicken skin begins to brown.

➤ Add the water and cover. Bring to a simmer, then reduce the heat to low and simmer for 10 to 15 minutes, skimming the top of the broth with a spoon as any foam or fat gathers. Turn the heat off and let it rest for 20 to 25 minutes, until the chicken is cooked through.

➤ Remove the chicken and discard the skin. Pull the meat from the bone and break into smaller pieces. Return meat to the pot. Add the pasta and the kale and warm over low heat for 1 to 2 minutes, stirring occasionally, until the kale is softened. Serve immediately.

PER SERVING (2 CUPS): 228 calories, 11 g protein, 34 g carbohydrates, 6 g fat (1 g saturated), 15 mg cholesterol, 5 g fiber, 465 mg sodium

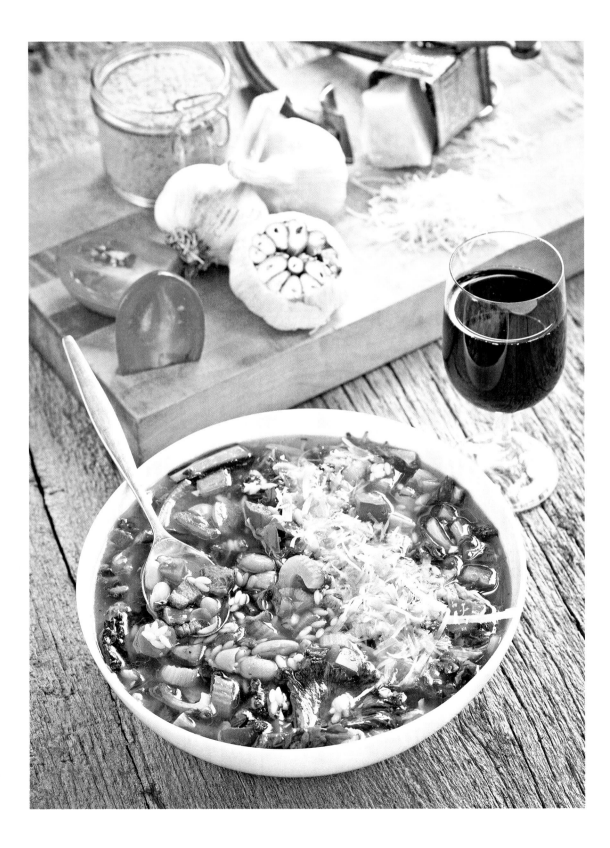

Pasta e Fagioli

This traditional Italian soup offers the best of both worlds: incredible flavor with serious nutrition. Every spoonful offers a little goodness and indulgence in the same bite—beans and bacon, kale and wine. High in protein and fiber but low in calories, it's a match made in heaven. **Serves 4**

½ cup dried pasta, such as small shells or orzo

1 tablespoon olive oil

2 slices nitrate-free bacon, chopped

½ teaspoon freshly ground black pepper

1 yellow onion, chopped

3 carrots, peeled and chopped

3 celery stalks, chopped

4 large garlic cloves, minced

4 cups Simple Chicken Broth (page 108)

1 cup dry white or red wine

1 pound ripe tomatoes, chopped (about 4 medium tomatoes)

One 15-ounce can navy or cannellini beans, drained and well rinsed

5 ounces kale, trimmed and cut into thin strips (about 5 cups)

¼ cup grated Parmesan cheese

➤ Cook the pasta for 2 minutes less than called for on the package instructions. Drain and set aside.

➤ Place the olive oil, bacon, and black pepper in a large saucepan over medium heat and cook for 4 to 5 minutes, until the bacon starts to crisp.

➤ Add the onion, carrots, celery, and garlic and cook for 2 to 3 minutes more, until the vegetables begin to soften. Add the chicken broth, wine, tomatoes, and beans. Bring to a simmer, then reduce the heat to medium-low and simmer for 10 to 15 minutes, until the vegetables are soft and the pasta is tender. Add the kale, reduce the heat to low, and cook for 2 minutes more, stirring often, until the kale is soft. Spoon into bowls, sprinkle with the cheese, and serve immediately.

PER SERVING (2 CUPS): 370 calories, 16 g protein, 48 g carbohydrates, 9 g fat (3 g saturated), 9 mg cholesterol, 9 g fiber, 770 mg sodium

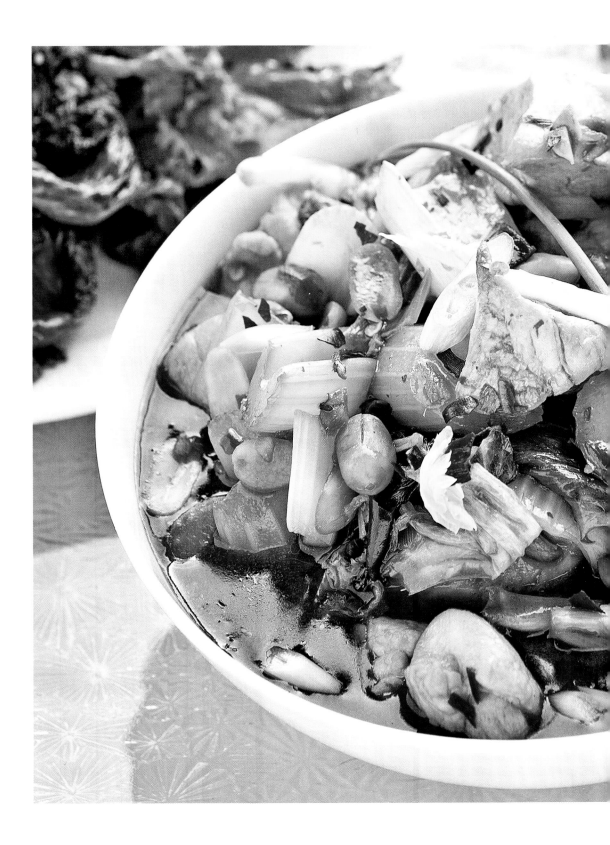

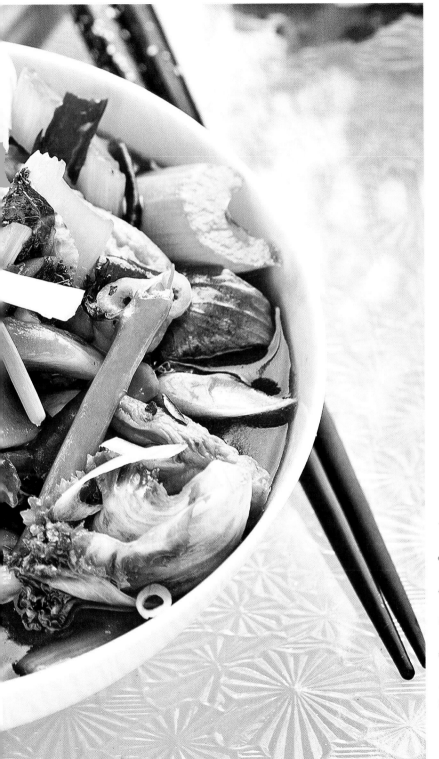

Kung
Pao
Chicken
with Kale

SEE PAGE 116

Kung Pao Chicken with Kale

If you like it hot, you've met your match. This healthy re-creation of the popular Chinese takeout dish delivers all of the lip-burning spice coveted by its devotees, minus the grease, MSG, and soaring sodium content. Try substituting almonds for the peanuts and get extra manganese, which can help promote healthy thyroid function and protect your cells from free radical damage. **Serves 4**

For the sauce

½ cup water

½ cup Simple Chicken Broth (page 108)

1 tablespoon light soy sauce

1 tablespoon brown sugar

1 tablespoon balsamic or black vinegar

2 teaspoons cornstarch

1 tablespoon canola oil

For the chicken

1 tablespoon cornstarch

2 tablespoons reduced-sodium soy sauce

2 tablespoons dry sherry

One 2-inch piece fresh ginger, chopped

2 garlic cloves, thinly sliced

1 teaspoon sesame oil

2 boneless, skinless chicken breasts, cut into ½-inch chunks

8 small dried red chiles, such as Sichuan or Arbol, chopped

Olive oil cooking spray

4 stalks celery, cut into ½-inch chunks

5 ounces kale, trimmed and chopped (about 5 cups)

2 tablespoons unsalted roasted peanuts

4 scallions, thinly sliced

2 cups cooked brown rice for serving

➤ Place all the ingredients for the sauce in a small bowl and whisk until smooth. Set aside.

➤ Place the cornstarch, 1 tablespoon of the soy sauce, the sherry, ginger, garlic, and sesame oil in a medium bowl. Whisk well to combine. Add the chicken and chiles and toss well to coat. Set aside.

➤ Heat a large skillet over high heat and coat it with cooking spray. Add the chicken, its marinade, the celery, and kale and cook for 1 to 2 minutes, stirring once or twice, until the chicken starts to brown. Add a little water if the chicken starts to stick.

➤ Reduce the heat to low and add the sauce. Cover and cook for 2 to 3 minutes, until the chicken is cooked through and the sauce thickens. Sprinkle with the scallions and serve immediately with the rice.

PER SERVING (2 CUPS): 405 calories, 31 g protein, 38 g carbohydrates, 10 g fat (1 g saturated), 72 mg cholesterol, 4 g fiber, 557 mg sodium

Did You Know? Commonly referred to as "MSG," monosodium glutamate is a food additive commonly found in Chinese food and some processed and canned foods. It is classified as "safe" by the FDA, but many people suffer adverse reactions to this "flavor enhancer," such as headaches and nausea, and it has even been linked to endocrine disruption and other health issues. When ordering from Chinese restaurants, always ask if the food has been prepared with MSG—and be vigilant when reading the labels of canned soups, deli meats, and condiments.

Kale, Sausage, and White Bean Soup

There's nothing more cozy than a steaming bowl of soup on a chilly day (well, besides a fire and a bearskin rug, maybe). This rustic soup combines spicy sausage, tender cannellini beans, and kale for a protein trifecta. **Serves 8**

2 links hot Italian pork sausage, cut into 1-inch chunks

1 tablespoon extra virgin olive oil

1 red onion, chopped

4 garlic cloves, sliced

One 10-ounce bunch kale, trimmed and chopped (about 10 cups)

2 quarts Simple Chicken Broth (page 108)

One 15-ounce can cannellini beans, drained and rinsed

1 tablespoon chopped fresh rosemary leaves

½ teaspoon fennel seeds

½ cup grated Parmesan cheese

➤ Place the sausage in a large saucepan over medium heat; drizzle with the olive oil and toss to combine. Increase the heat to high and cook, stirring, until browned, about 4 minutes. Add the onion and cook for 3 to 4 minutes, until it starts to soften. Add the garlic and cook, stirring often, until fragrant, about 1 minute. Toss in the kale and stir to combine. Add the chicken broth and bring the mixture to a boil. Reduce the heat to low, cover, and simmer for 15 to 17 minutes, until the liquid has slightly decreased and the broth is flavored by the sausage.

➤ Add the beans, rosemary, and fennel seeds and stir to combine. Cook for 1 to 2 minutes to warm the beans. Serve immediately sprinkled with the cheese.

PER SERVING (2½ CUPS): 194 calories, 11 g protein, 22 g carbohydrates, 8 g fat (2 g saturated), 12 mg cholesterol, 5 g fiber, 577 mg sodium

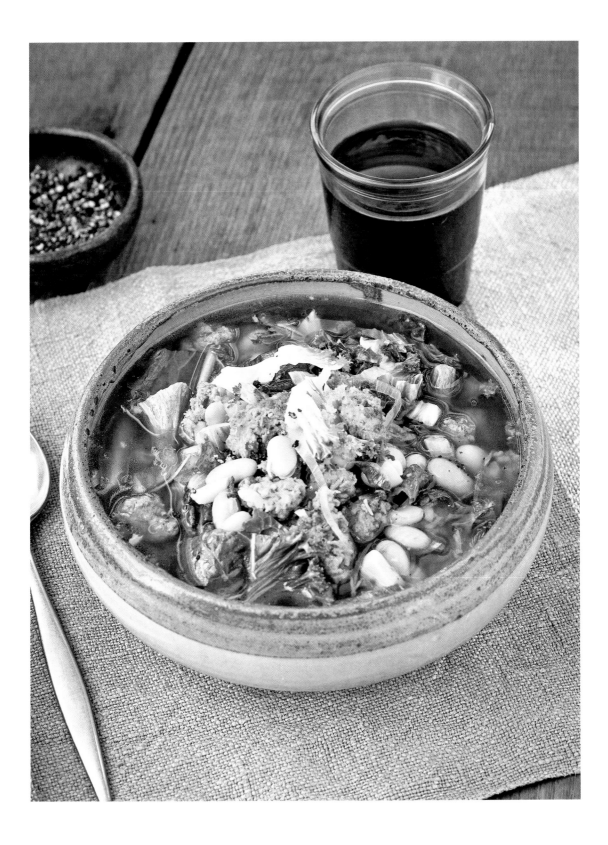

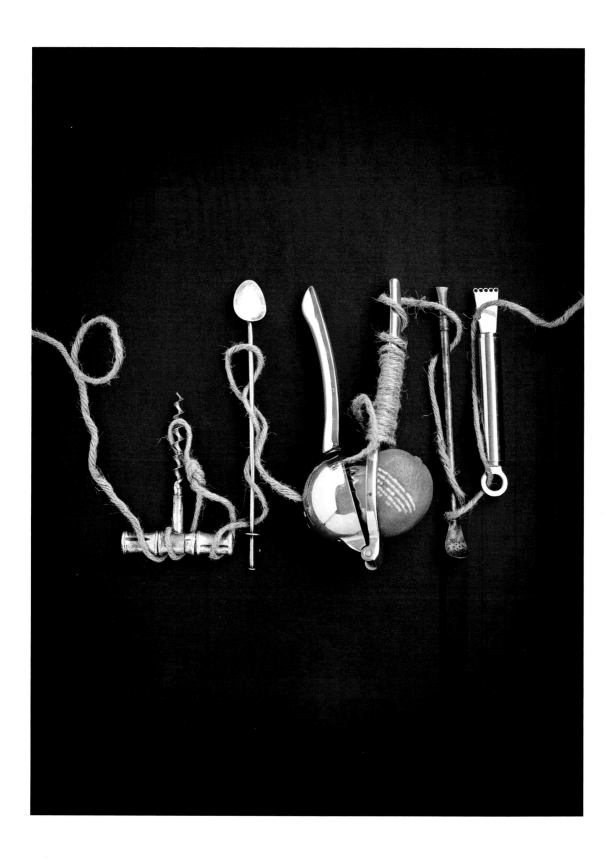

6.

Naughty and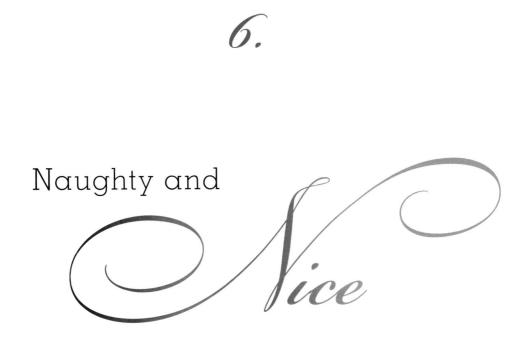

Kale Pisco Sour

One of Latin America's signature cocktails, the pisco sour was invented by an American bartender in the 1920s in Lima, Peru, and soon became a worldwide sensation. The lime juice and pisco liquor give this drink a unique tanginess that masks any "vegetable" flavor you might expect from the kale. This low-carb cocktail is Latin love at first sip. **Serves 4**

2 teaspoons granulated sugar

4 ounces pisco liquor

1 cup packed torn kale leaves

¼ cup packed mint leaves

¼ cup fresh lime juice

1 egg white

1 cup cold water

4 lime wedges

➤ Place all the ingredients except for the lime wedges in a blender. Add the cold water and blend on high speed until the kale is chopped and a thick foam forms on top. Transfer to 4 highball glasses and top each with a wedge of lime. Serve immediately.

PER SERVING (1 CUP): 172 calories, 2 g protein, 9 g carbohydrates, 0 g fat (0 g saturated), 0 mg cholesterol, 1 g fiber, 37 mg sodium

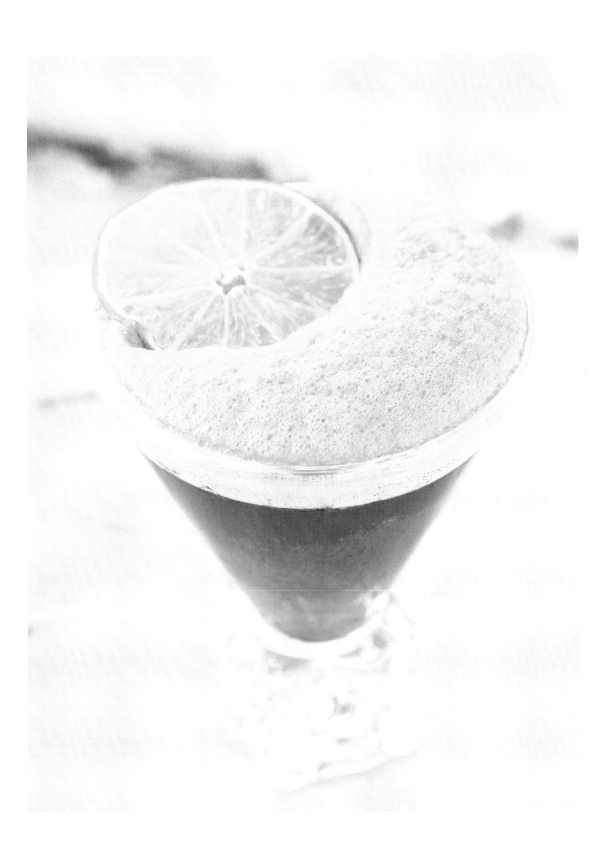

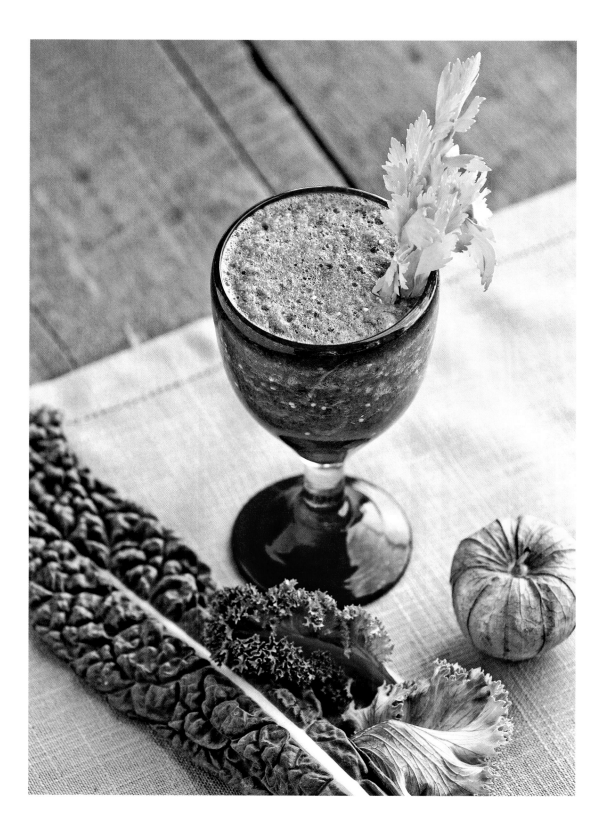

Green Bloody Mary

In this twist on everyone's favorite brunch drink, kale truly bleeds green. The addition of kale and whole tomatillos fortifies this savory drink with extra fiber and complex carbs, promoting a slow burn conducive to a relaxing, guilt-free afternoon.

Serves 2

4 tomatillos

½ cup packed torn kale leaves

½ small cucumber, peeled and quartered

Juice of ½ lemon

4 ounces vodka

1 tablespoon hot sauce

1 teaspoon Worcestershire sauce

¼ teaspoon celery salt

2 celery stalks for garnish

2 dashes Sriracha chili sauce, optional

➤ Bring a small saucepan of water to a boil. Add the tomatillos and cook for 3 to 4 minutes, until their skin softens. Drain and peel. Discard the peels and place the pulp in a blender along with the kale, cucumber, lemon juice, vodka, hot sauce, Worcestershire sauce, and celery salt. Blend until smooth. Transfer to 2 glasses filled with ice and garnish with the celery stalks. Add the Sriracha, if using. Serve immediately.

PER SERVING (1 CUP): 181 calories, 2 g protein, 10 g carbohydrates, 1 g fat (0 g saturated), 0 mg cholesterol, 3 g fiber, 487 mg sodium

Cherry Kale Campari

This simple, refreshing, low-alcohol drink is the perfect aperitif. Juicy black cherries not only balance the bitterness of the Campari, but their low glycemic index may also help regulate your blood sugar level, keeping hunger at bay. Cherries also contain potassium, which can help control blood pressure. And you'll need all the help you can get after indulging in a few of these with your paramour. . . . **Serves 2**

1½ cups frozen pitted black cherries

½ cup packed torn kale leaves

4 ounces Campari

4 ice cubes

4 small kale leaves, such as Red Russian

➤ Place the cherries, kale, Campari, and ice cubes in a blender and blend until smooth. Pour into 2 chilled glasses and serve immediately with the kale garnish.

PER SERVING (1 CUP): 213 calories, 1 g protein, 29 g carbohydrates, 0 g fat (0 g saturated), 0 mg cholesterol, 2 g fiber, 9 mg sodium

Did You Know? Campari is a type of Italian bitters distilled from a secret blend of herbs. The drink was supposedly invented around 1920 in Florence by bartender Luca Picchi and Count Camillo Negroni, after whom the Negroni cocktail (a classic, Campari-containing concoction) is named.

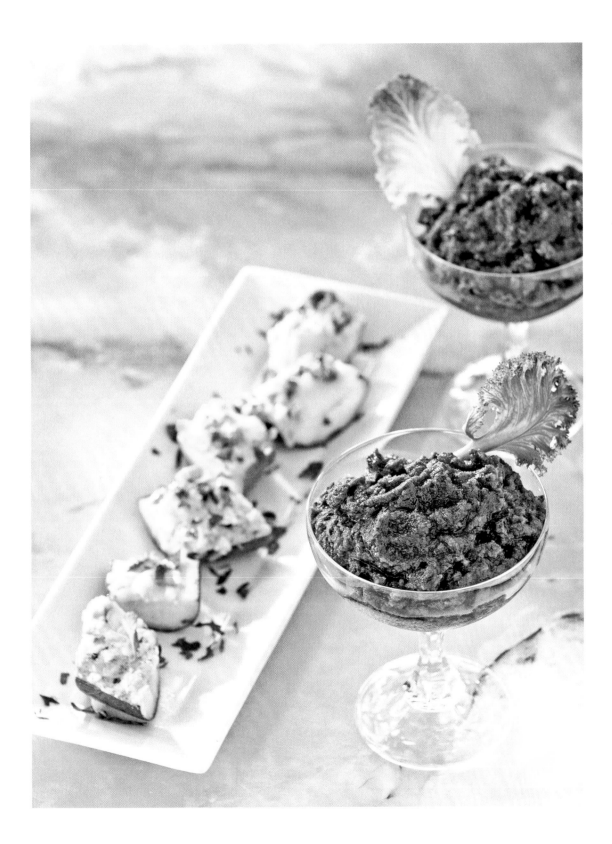

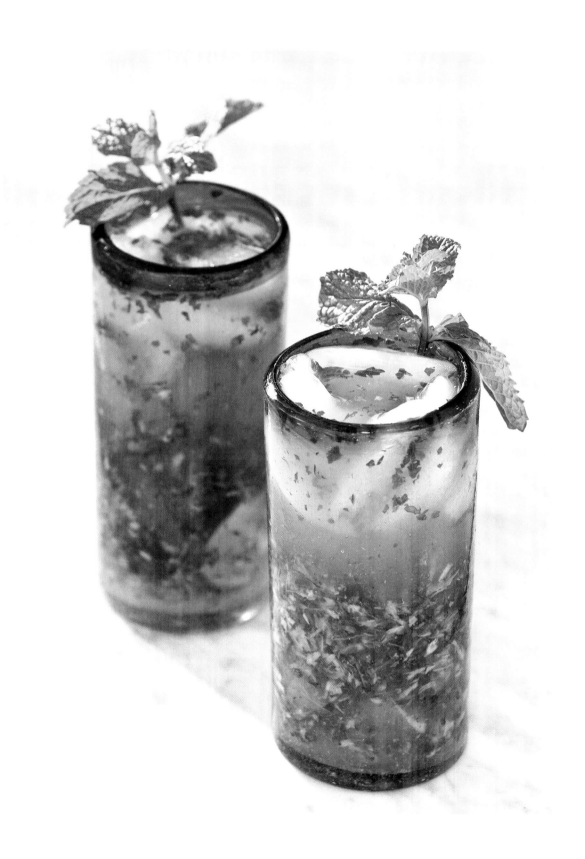

Kalejito

This cocktail's refreshing zing comes from a healthy dose of mint—an herb thought to relieve stress, aid digestion . . . and stimulate the senses. The addition of fresh kale intensifies its already vibrant green color, making for an elegant, gemlike cocktail that couldn't be more seductive. **Serves 2**

2 teaspoons superfine sugar

4 ounces white rum

½ cup packed torn kale leaves

½ cup packed mint leaves, plus 2 sprigs for garnish

Juice of 2 limes (about ¼ cup)

➤ Combine all the ingredients in a blender and blend on high speed. Pour over 2 glasses filled with ice. Garnish with the mint sprigs and serve immediately.

PER SERVING (1 CUP): 179 calories, 1 g protein, 13 g carbohydrates, 0 g fat (0 g saturated), 0 mg cholesterol, 2 g fiber, 16 mg sodium

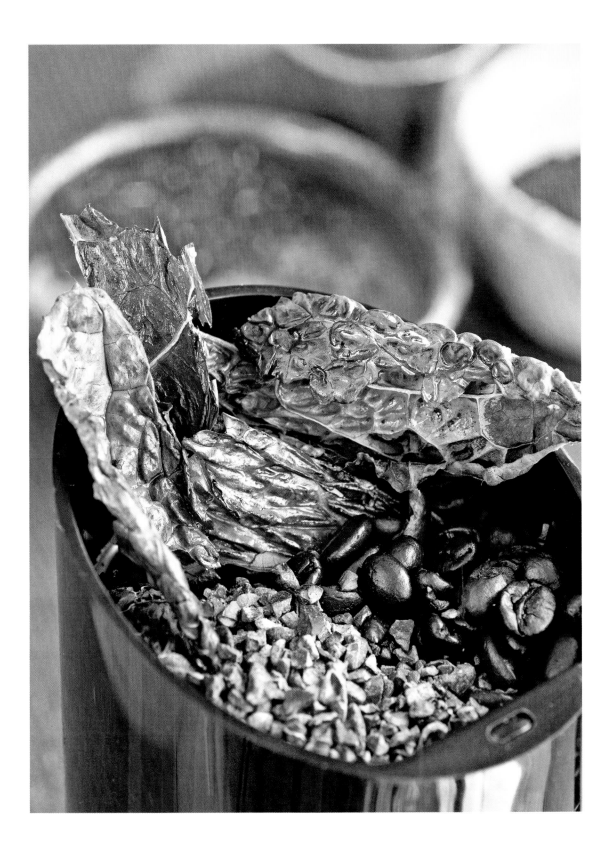

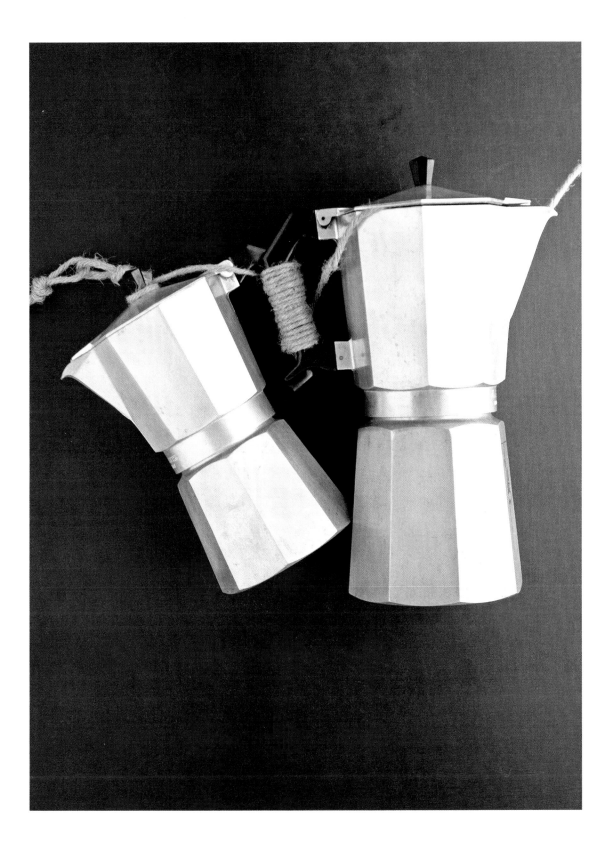

The Lacchiato

Throw on a robe and surprise your love with the perfect morning pick-me-up. More impressive than a coffee shop macchiato is this kale "lacchiato," made with leftover kale chips ground to a fine powder and mixed with coffee beans and cacao nibs. What happens when you combine these three superfoods—is this the Viagra of the natural world? We'll let you be the judge. **Serves 2**

1½ tablespoons dark roasted coffee beans

2 teaspoons cacao nibs

2–3 medium-sized Roasted Kale Chips (page 42)

¼ cup whole milk

➤ Place the coffee beans, cacao nibs, and large kale chip in a coffee grinder. Grind until finely ground. Follow your coffee machine's instructions to brew one serving of coffee. Heat the milk and froth it, if desired. Divide the coffee between 2 cups and top each with half of the hot milk. Place the small kale chip in the coffee grinder and finely grind it. Sprinkle over the lacchiatos and serve immediately.

PER SERVING (1 LACCHIATO): 44 calories, 1 g protein, 2 g carbohydrates, 3 g fat (1 g saturated), 3 mg cholesterol, 0 g fiber, 17 mg sodium

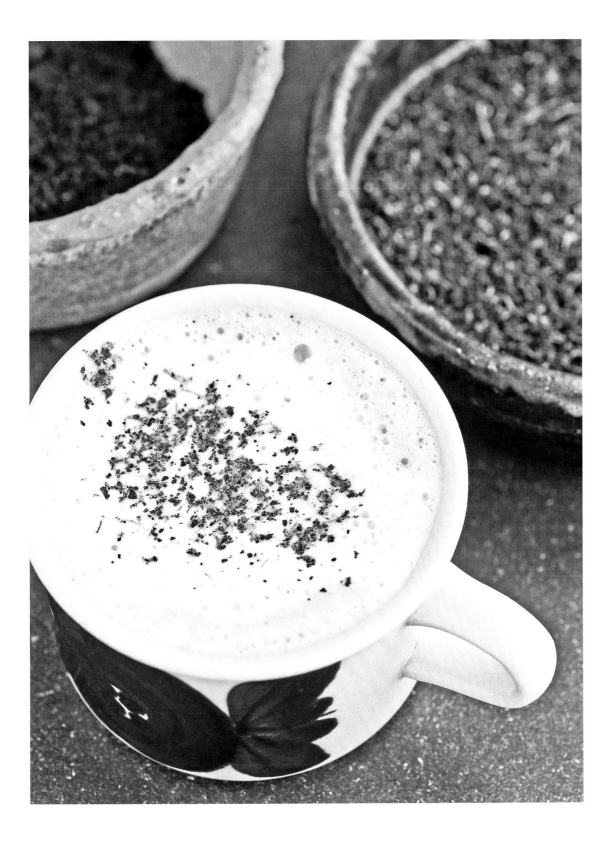

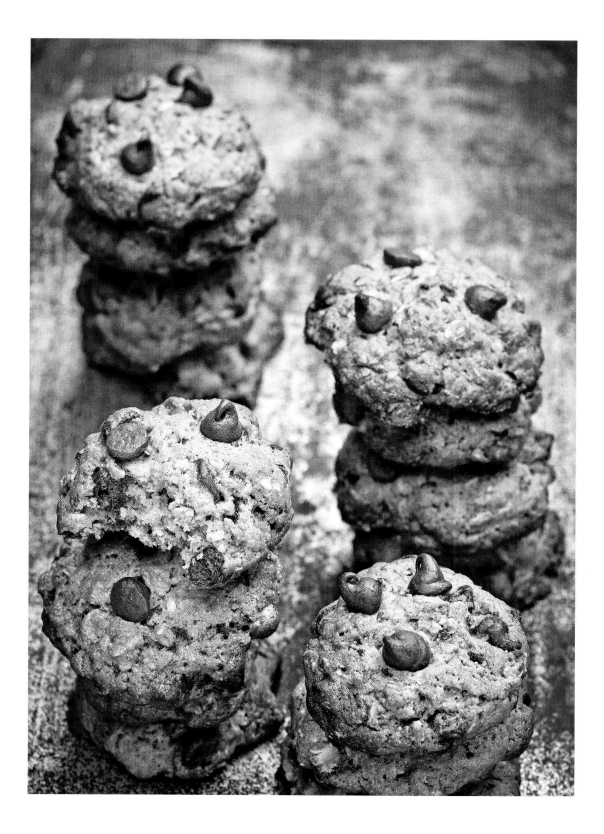

Chocolate Chip Kale Cookies

You smell it, you crave it, you must have it. Who can resist the siren song of chocolate chip cookies fresh from the oven? This nutritious batch is made with whole wheat pastry flour and oats, spiked with a small hit of kale. Don't forget to let them cool before indulging . . . you wouldn't want to get burned by temptation. **Makes 24 cookies**

Nonstick cooking spray

1¼ cups white whole wheat or pastry flour

½ cup old-fashioned oats

2 teaspoons baking powder

¼ teaspoon salt

½ cup packed torn kale leaves

1 cup firmly packed light brown sugar

½ cup (1 stick) unsalted butter, softened

1 tablespoon molasses

2 large eggs

1 tablespoon vanilla extract (or substitute ¼ teaspoon mint extract)

1 cup 70% cocoa semisweet chocolate chips (or 70% cocoa dark chocolate chunks)

➤ Preheat the oven to 350°F and coat 2 baking sheets with cooking spray.

➤ Place the flour, oats, baking powder and salt in a large bowl and stir well. Set aside.

➤ Place the kale in a food processor and pulse 10 to 15 times, until it is finely chopped but not pureed. Place the brown sugar and butter in a large bowl and beat with an electric mixer on low speed until thoroughly combined. Add the molasses and eggs, one at a time, mixing on low speed until just incorporated. Add the vanilla extract and mix until well combined. Slowly add the dry ingredients, mixing to combine.

➤ Add the chocolate chips and stir with a wooden spoon 2 or 3 times to distribute. Using a tablespoon, drop the batter onto the greased baking sheet, each dropful about 1 inch apart. (You will need to make the cookies in batches.) Bake for 12 to 14 minutes, until the cookies are firm around the edges but still slightly soft in the center. Transfer the cookies to a wire rack to cool completely.

PER SERVING (1 COOKIE): 141 calories, 1 g protein, 19 g carbohydrates, 7 g fat (4 g saturated), 16 mg cholesterol, 0.4 g fiber, 54 mg sodium

Kale and Black Cherry Sorbet

This low-cal sorbet is cool, dark, rich, and handsome . . . what's not to like? And at less than 100 calories per serving, you can indulge in a double scoop without burdening your conscience (or your waistline). Garnish with a little fresh thyme—which adds a nice herbaceous quality—or mint for a clean, refreshing finish. Serves 8

2 cups frozen pitted black cherries, plus 8 cherries for garnish

½ cup packed torn kale leaves, stems removed

4 ounces almond-flavored liqueur

2 cups water

8 sprigs fresh thyme or mint for garnish

➤ Place all the ingredients in a blender and blend until smooth. Transfer to an ice cream maker and process according to the manufacturer's instructions. Or freeze in an airtight container for at least 4 hours. Defrost for 5 to 10 minutes on the countertop before serving. Garnish with the reserved cherries and thyme.

PER SERVING (½ CUP): 82 calories, 1 g protein, 6 g carbohydrates, 0 g fat (0 g saturated), 0 mg cholesterol, 1 g fiber, 5 mg sodium

Did You Know? In the Middle Ages, women gave knights and warriors gifts that included thyme leaves before their men headed off to battle. They believed thyme would bring courage to their paramours, and it can bring flavor and good health to you. Thyme is high in iron, and like most herbs has natural antibacterial compounds that can ward off illness.

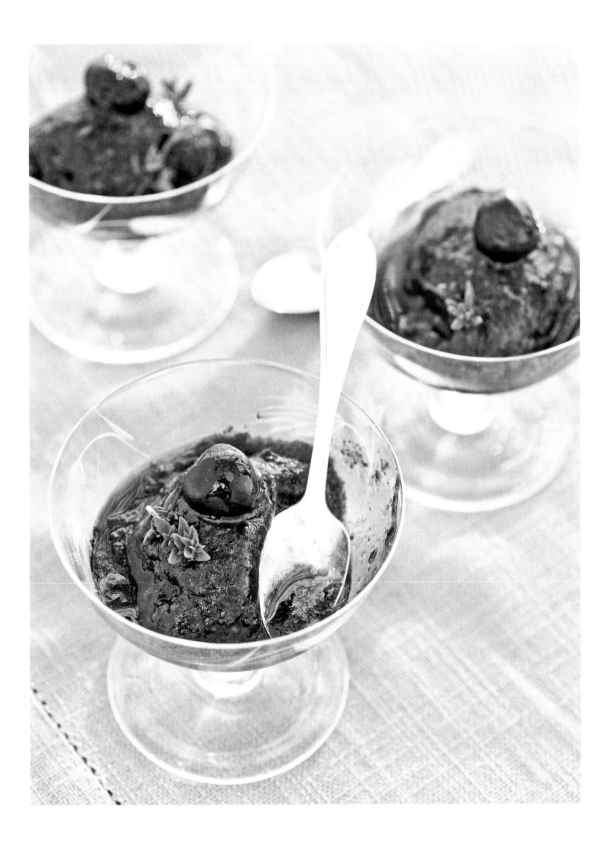

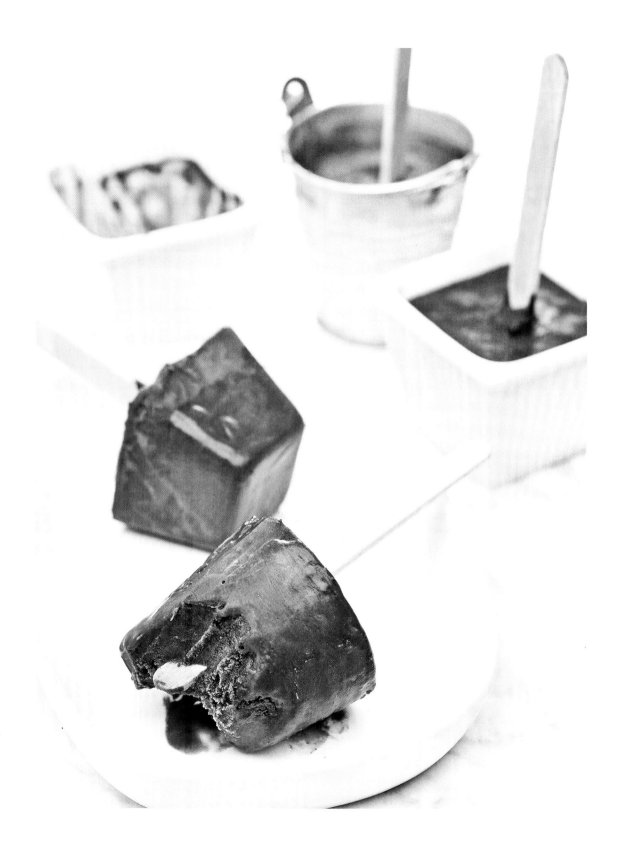

Chocolate Kale Fudge Pops

These rich, indulgent fudge pops get a boost of fiber thanks to a hearty dose of kale. You might not think of fiber as sexy, but getting adequate fiber can lead to flatter abs and clearer skin. Fiber also helps to maintain the balance of healthy bacteria in your intestinal tract, which promotes immunity and can even enhance your libido. Seconds, anyone? **Serves 8**

1 cup granulated sugar

1 cup unsweetened cocoa powder

1 teaspoon vanilla extract

½ teaspoon ground cinnamon

⅛ teaspoon ground nutmeg

⅛ teaspoon ground coriander

2 cups warm water

1 cup torn kale leaves

➤ In a large saucepan, combine all ingredients except the kale and add the warm water. Bring to a boil, then reduce the heat and simmer for 2 to 3 minutes, stirring occasionally, until the mixture is smooth and thick. Remove from the heat and cool to room temperature. Place the kale in a food processor and pulse until finely chopped. Stir the kale into the chocolate mixture and divide it among 8 ice pop molds and insert ice pop sticks.

➤ Freeze for at least 4 hours before serving. The pops will keep for up to 3 weeks in an airtight container in the freezer.

PER SERVING (1 POP): 127 calories, 2 g protein, 32 g carbohydrates, 1 g fat (1 g saturated), 0 mg cholesterol, 4 g fiber, 8 mg sodium

Dark Tropical Kiss

Some couples were just meant to be together . . . and sweet, flaky coconut enrobed by dark, bittersweet chocolate is simply a match made in heaven. In addition to a buzz-worthy collection of natural stimulants, cacao is a great source of flavonoid antioxidants, iron, and manganese, all needed by the brain to produce and enjoy a remarkable kiss. **Serves 4**

Nonstick cooking spray

6 tablespoons superfine sugar

1 large egg white

½ cup sweetened shredded coconut

¼ cup unsweetened cacao nibs

One 10-ounce bunch kale, trimmed and torn into 4-inch-wide pieces

➤ Preheat the oven to 300°F and coat 3 baking sheets with the nonstick cooking spray.

➤ In a large bowl, combine the sugar and egg white. Using a whisk, beat the sugar into the egg until frothy, about 1 minute.

➤ Spread out the coconut and cacao nibs on a piece of waxed paper or a plate and mix them together with your fingertips.

➤ Dip the edges of the kale leaves into the egg white mixture. Press the egg-covered edges into the coconut-cacao mixture. Place on the baking sheets and bake for 10 to 14 minutes, until the kale is crisp and the coconut is lightly browned. Serve immediately.

PER SERVING (2 CUPS): 240 calories, 4 g protein, 34 g carbohydrates, 10 g fat (7 g saturated), 0 mg cholesterol, 3 g fiber, 74 mg sodium

Did You Know? Chocolate contains an alkaloid molecule called theobromine. In humans, its effect is similar to that of caffeine (on a smaller scale). But in animals, theobromine can cause wild heart palpitations, which is why dogs should never eat chocolate.

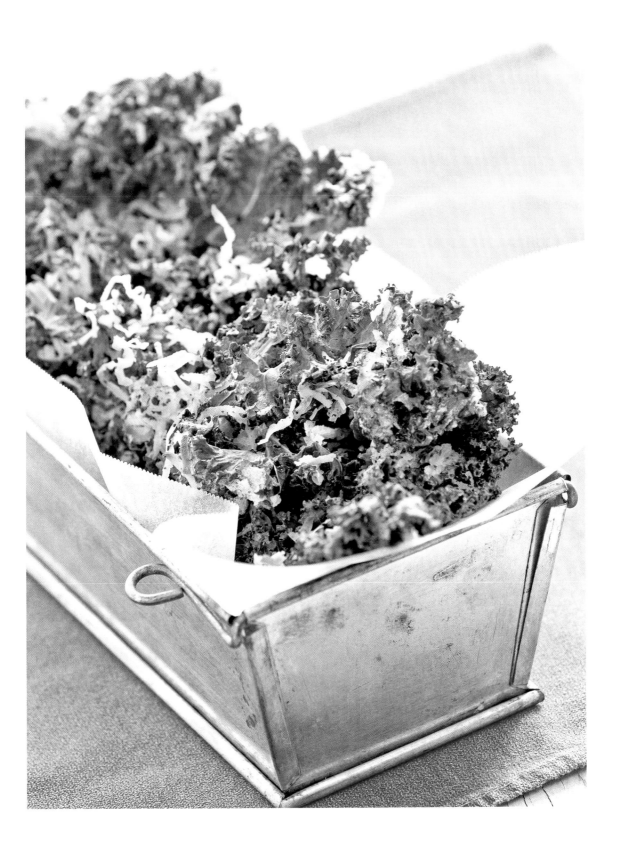

Party with Your Girl

Quick Kale Dips and Spreads

Looking to add more life to your party? Kale is so versatile and agreeable that it's easy to take her anywhere—she blends in perfectly. Prep her for any party by washing her squeaky clean, patting her dry, and then finely chopping her in a food processor. Here are a few ways to add kale to your favorite party mix.

Kale Artichoke Dip

Put a fresh spin on your favorite recipe for spinach artichoke dip and substitute equal portions of finely chopped fresh kale. While you're at it, you can also swap out the mayo for Kale-onaise (page 53).

Baked Kale and Brie

Add a little nutrition to this much-loved appetizer by skipping the puff pastry and dressing your cheese with a pretty layer of kale! Preheat the oven to 350°F. Cut off the top rind of an 8-inch wheel of brie and press ¼ cup chopped dried cherries and 1 cup of finely chopped kale into the cheese. Place the brie on a sheet pan lined with parchment paper, and bake 5 to 7 minutes for a deliciously gooey treat. Serve with plain, crisp crackers.

Hot Kale Crab Dip

Follow your own tried-and-true crab dip recipe but before baking, fold in 1 cup of finely chopped kale (you can also use kale to replace the parsley). Serve with crudité or whole wheat crackers.

Pesto Hummus

Make a Kale Drizzle by combining kale, olive oil, and salt in a food processor (see Green Pizza recipe, page 80). Spoon a little over store-bought hummus and serve with baked pita chips.

Kale Ranch Dip

Blend 1 cup of sour cream with your favorite Ranch-style seasoning, and stir in 1 cup of finely chopped kale for a heartier and healthier dip. Serve with a variety of fresh veggies or Kale Chips (page 42).

Lemony Kale Shrimp Dip

Combine 1 cup of Kale-onaise (page 53) to ½ pound peeled and deveined fresh or frozen shrimp (if using frozen, allow to thaw). Pulse shrimp in a food processor to roughly chop before blending with Kale-onaise. Serve with lemon wedges and a bottle of your favorite hot sauce on the side, and small rye toasts for dipping.

Kale Romesco

Romesco is a Spanish sauce made with roasted red peppers, garlic, olive oil, and nuts. It's even more delicious (and pretty) when you add in a cup of chopped kale. You can serve it over practically anything, from fish to chicken. It also makes a great party dip with fresh veggies or crackers on the side.

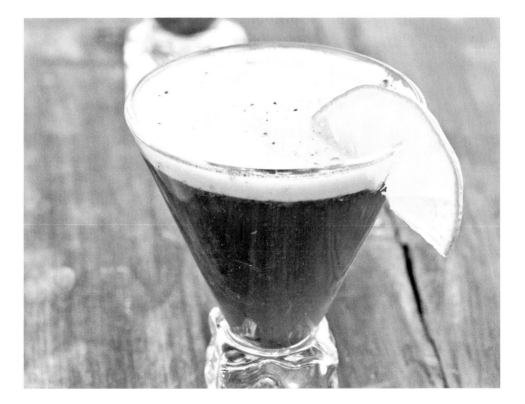

Metric Conversion Chart

Oven Temperature Equivalents

250 °F = 120 °C	275 °F = 135 °C
300 °F = 150 °C	325 °F = 160 °C
350 °F = 180 °C	375 °F = 190 °C
400 °F = 200 °C	425 °F = 220 °C
450 °F = 230 °C	475 °F = 240 °C
500 °F = 260 °C	

Liquid Ingredients

The United States traditionally uses cup measures for liquid and solid ingredients, and spoon measures for smaller amounts of ingredients. Measurements should always be level unless directed otherwise.

⅛ teaspoon = 0.5 mL	¼ teaspoon = 1 mL
½ teaspoon = 2 mL	1 teaspoon = 5 mL
1 tablespoon = 3 teaspoons = ½ fluid ounce = 15 mL	2 tablespoons = ⅓ cup = 1 fluid ounce = 30 mL
4 tablespoons = ¼ cup = 2 fluid ounces = 60 mL	5⅓ tablespoons = ⅛ cup = 3 fluid ounces = 80 mL
8 tablespoons = ½ cup = 4 fluid ounces = 120 mL	10⅔ tablespoons = ⅔ cup = 5 fluid ounces = 160 mL
12 tablespoons = ¾ cup = 6 fluid ounces = 180 mL	16 tablespoons = 1 cup = 8 fluid ounces = 240 mL

1 pint = 2 cups = 16 fluid ounces = 480 mL	1 quart = 4 cups = 32 fluid ounces = 960 mL

Dry Ingredients

½ ounce = 15 g	1 ounce = 30 g
4 ounces (¼ pound) = 120 g	8 ounces (½ pound) = 240 g
16 ounces (1 pound) = 480 g	

Conversion by Ingredient

*S*tandard cup measurements for solid and dry ingredients will vary in weight based on the ingredient, while cup measurements for liquids are always the same (independent of ingredient).

STANDARD CUP	FINE POWDER (FLOUR)	GRAIN (RICE)	GRANULAR (SUGAR)	LIQUID SOLIDS (BUTTER)	LIQUIDS (WATER)
⅛	18 g	19 g	24 g	25 g	30 mL
¼	35 g	38 g	48 g	50 g	60 mL
⅓	47 g	50 g	63 g	67 g	80 mL
½	70 g	75 g	95 g	100 g	120 mL
⅔	93 g	100 g	125 g	133 g	160 mL
¾	105 g	113 g	143 g	150 g	180 mL
1	140 g	150 g	190 g	200 g	240 mL

Miscellaneous

1 medium carrot (3 ounces, 7 inches) = ½ cup	1 red or green bell pepper (5 ounces) = ½ heaping cup
1 22 ounce head broccoli = 4 cups	1 small head of romaine = 6 ounces (3 cups)
1 cup grated cheddar cheese (1 ¾ ounce)	1 red onion = 2 cups chopped = 14 ounces
1 link fresh chorizo or Italian sausage = 3 ounces, about 1 cup chopped	1 jalapeno = ¼ cup ounces, 1.5 ounces
1 cup chopped kale = 1 ounce	1 cup frozen cherries = 4 ½ ounces
1 kiwi = 2 ounces ⅓ cup	1 lime juiced = 2 tablespoons
¼ cup cilantro = .5 ounces	4 scallions = ¼ cup = 1.5 ounces
2 stalks celery = 4/14 ounces, 1 cup	

Get Sneaky with Her

*O*nce you're hooked on kale, you'll want to flirt with her throughout the day and find ways to sneak her into every meal. Here are some tricky ways to get a dose of nutrition, even when you don't have a lot time to cook.

Order In with Her

Gotta have your Chinese takeout fix? Instead of loading up on white rice, use washed kale leaves to wrap handfuls of your meal and munch away. No plates or chopsticks required.

Sandwich Her

Season kale leaves with a teaspoon of olive oil and a pinch of salt. Tuck the leaves between two slices of whole wheat bread, then layer on your favorite fixins' for a satisfying sandwich that doesn't skimp on greens.

Don't Leave Home Without Her

Before you leave for work, chop two kale leaves in the food processor and transfer to a small resealable bag. Stir your handy bag of kale into takeout soups, chili, and stews to increase the portion size and nutrition of your desk lunch.

Supercharge Your Pizza

Thinly slice kale into ribbons and dress with a teaspoon of olive oil and salt. Store in the fridge while you're waiting for the pizza delivery boy (or while making your own). When you're ready to dig into a delicious slice, sprinkle a handful of kale on top.

Go Mile-High

Nothing cramps your style, your health, or your taste buds more than airplane food. Pack your own kale salad, or bring a baggie of Kale Chips (page 42) to munch on in lieu of mystery meat or salted peanuts. Your body will thank you when you deplane.

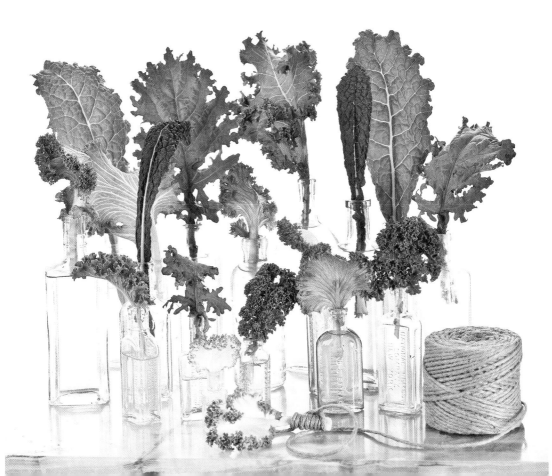

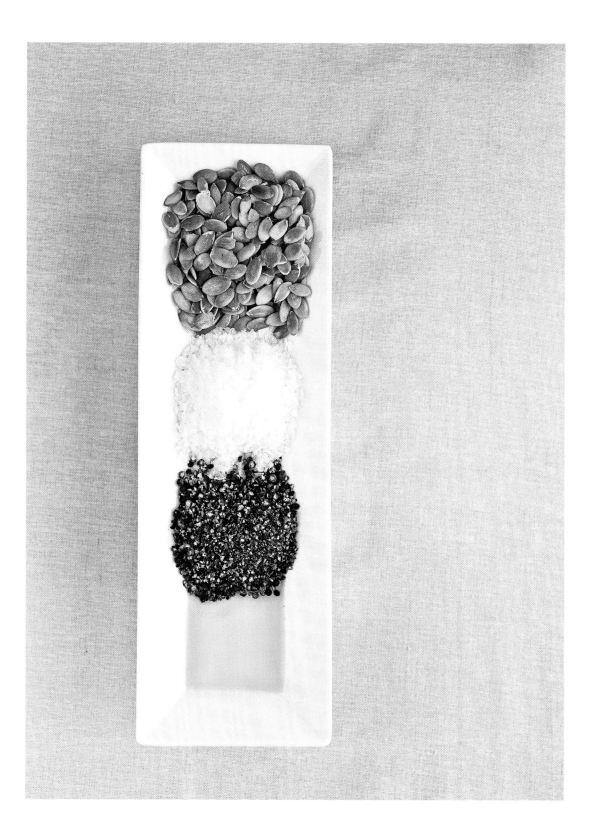

Resources

$\mathcal{S}$hred pounds, boost libido, and save the economy. Buying local food is one of the best ways to contribute to your community. Your food dollars help support farmers who are farming responsibly and raising animals in a humane and sustainable way. Here are some resources for finding the high-quality ingredients recommended in this book.

Grass-Fed Beef and Pork

www.eatwild.com
www.localharvest.org
www.americangrass-fed.org
www.organicprairie.com
www.hardwickbeef.com
www.fleishers.com
www.dicksonsfarmstand.com
www.sugarmtnfarm.com
www.texasgrass-fedbeef.com/id55.htm

Eggs

www.naturesyoke.com
www.peteandgerrys.com

Local Dairy and Grass-fed Dairy

www.ronnybrook.com
www.pastureland.coop/buy/direct
www.grass-fedtraditions.com/grass
   _fed_butter.htm
www.kerrygold.com/products

And for More Kale-rotica:

www.kalecrusaders.com/p/about-us
   .html
thekaleproject.com
kaleuniversity.org/3901-learn-local
   -farms-farmers-markets
www.grownyc.org/greenmarket
foodcoop.com

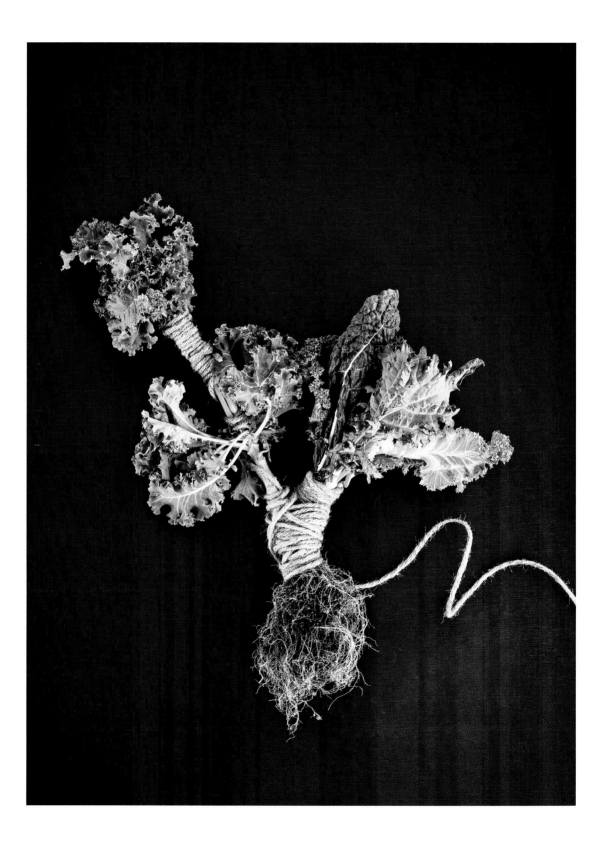

Acknowledgments

We set out to share our love and enjoyment of kale, and have had tremendous fun producing this book for you. Gratitude, praise, and recognition to the following people who have been part of our journey:

Karen Rinaldi and Julie Will and their team at HarperWave provided the perfect polish to take our love of kale and create the beautiful book you hold.

A big thanks to Uli Iserloh and his team at Bright Launch, who expertly managed production of this project initially as an e-book. As a digital marketing mastermind, Uli was also responsible for the launch of our website and social media efforts.

Many thanks to Joy Tutela and the David Black Agency for their guidance on this project and consistent encouragement and support. Joy has an incredibly sharp eye, wit, and business savvy. She has guided us through the world of publishing with a kind and steady hand. Words cannot express our gratitude.

We are grateful for the long hours, dedication, and great eye that Ian McSpadden brought to the set shooting the photographs and to Mutual Endeavours Farm for hosting. Thanks, Jerry and Catherine, who were our lifeline during the shoot and our favorite taste testers.

Finally, a heartfelt thanks to the countless readers of our previous books, *Secrets of a Skinny Chef* and *The Happiness Diet,* as well as the readers on our Recipe for Happiness and Skinny Chef blogs—sharing their precious insights, comments, feedback, and stories to enrich the community of healthy eaters and cooks.

At the core of it, food should be celebrated, appreciated, and shared every day with friends and family, and we are excited to share this book and its fifty delicious, nutritious dishes with you.

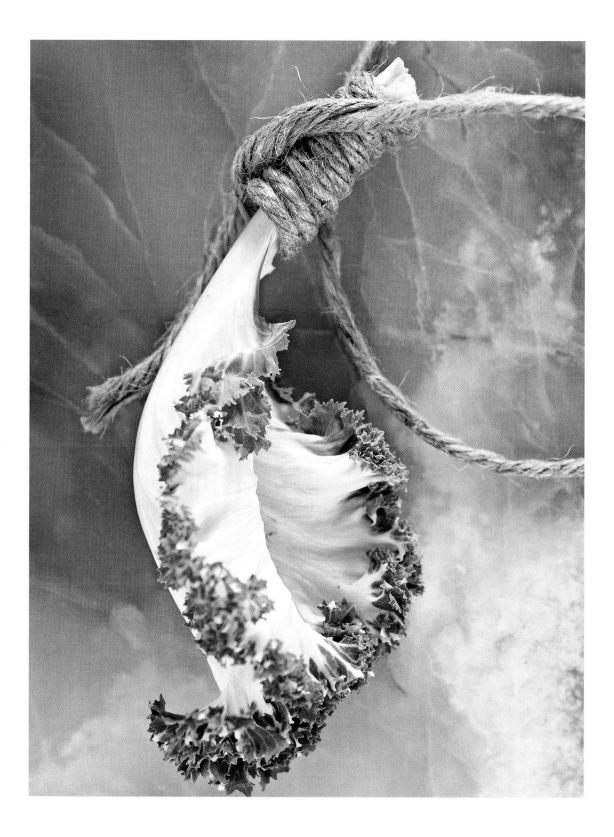

Index

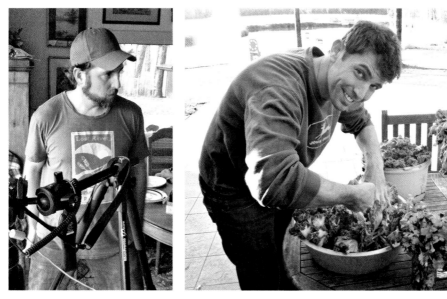

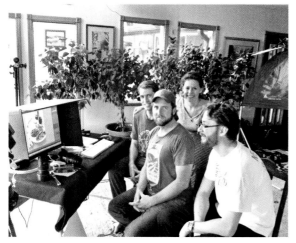

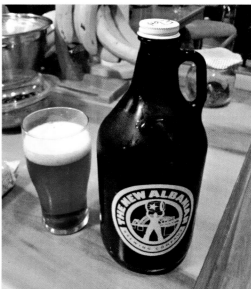

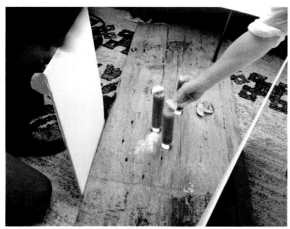

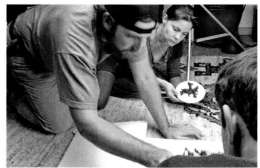

About the Authors

Drew Ramsey, M.D., is a psychiatrist, author, and farmer. He is one of psychiatry's leading proponents of using dietary change to help balance moods, sharpen brain function, and improve mental health. His clinical work focuses on the treatment of depression and anxiety with a combination of psychotherapy, lifestyle modification, and psychopharmacology.

Dr. Ramsey is an assistant clinical professor of psychiatry at Columbia University in New York and an attending psychiatrist at the New York State Psychiatric Institute. He is a diplomate of the American Board of Psychiatry and Neurology and completed his specialty training in adult psychiatry at Columbia University/New York State Psychiatric Institute. He earned his M.D. from Indiana University School of Medicine and is a Phi Beta Kappa graduate of Earlham College.

Dr. Ramsey regularly provides information and opinion on psychiatry-related topics in the media. His writing and commentary have appeared in publications such as the *New York Times*, the *Wall Street Journal*, the *Atlantic*, and *Men's Journal* and he has appeared on CBS News, *The Doctors*, and NPR, among other outlets. He is also the coauthor of *The Happiness Diet* and regularly blogs for DrewRamseyMD.com and PsychologyToday.com. He lives in New York City with his wife and daughter.

Jennifer Iserloh believes that the essence of good health springs from your own kitchen. She is the author of *Secrets of a Skinny Chef, Yoga Body Diet*, and *Active Calorie Diet*. As a trained chef, Jennifer has created thousands of delicious recipes, articles, for broadcast and print media, including *Today,*